# Concise N

# Other Examination Preparation Books Published by Petroc Press:

# Concise Notes in Oncology

**Kefah M. Mokbel** MB, BS (Lond.), FRCS (Eng.), FRCS (Gen.)

*Department of Surgery*
*Northwick Park and St Mark's Hospitals*
*Harrow, Middlesex, UK*

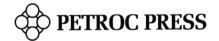 **PETROC PRESS**

*Petroc Press,* an imprint of LibraPharm Limited

**Distributors**

Plymbridge Distributors Limited, Plymbridge House, Estover Road, Plymouth PL6 7PZ, UK

Published in the United Kingdom by LibraPharm Limited, 3b Thames Court, High Street, Goring-on-Thames, Reading, Berks RG8 9AQ

A catalogue record for this book is available from the British Library

ISBN 1 900603 46 2

Printed and bound in the United Kingdom by
MPG Books Limited, Bodmin, Cornwall PL31 1EG

# Contents

# Foreword

The management of patients diagnosed with cancer is an ever changing and, fortunately, an improving field. Of course, patients initially present with a variety of symptoms, but only the minority actually prove to have an underlying malignancy as the cause for these symptoms. In the first instance most are referred for assessment and investigations by their general practitioners to a surgeon with an appropriate regional subspecialty interest. Once the diagnosis of cancer has been established, the treatment is increasingly becoming multidisciplinary, with more patients needing combination treatment under the care of a multidisciplinary specialist team, including surgeon, oncologist and well-trained support staff.

The optimal management of patients with cancer relies on an up-to-date understanding of not only the treatment options, but also the underlying rationale for such treatment and the tumour biology upon which these are based. *Concise Notes in Oncology* is a brief but detailed up-to-date summary of major components of modern oncological care. It gives an excellent outline of basic tumour biology and provides an easily accessible, well-organised summary of optimal oncological patient management classified by tumour type. I feel that this book will be an invaluable aid to all those working in this field, but especially junior doctors preparing for their membership and fellow examinations, general practitioners and clinical nurse specialists. By its very nature, this book is brief, but this is one of the advantages as this makes for easy access and use. Due to the ever-changing field of oncology, *Concise Notes in Oncology* will of course need regular review and updating, but its format and style should make this relatively straightforward and I am confident that it will provide an invaluable aid to other more detailed and extensive oncology texts.

*January, 1998*                    Nigel P. M. Sacks, MS, FRCS, FRACS
Consultant Surgeon
The Royal Marsden and St George's Hospitals
London

# Preface

This book has two objectives. It is intended to provide an accurate, concise source of information in medical and surgical oncology and to serve as a platform on which to build new information as generated by the multitude of scientific and clinical disciplines which continuously contribute to improving our understanding of cancer and its management.

Each cancer is presented in an organised format which includes information about epidemiology, aetiology, pathology, clinical features, investigations, treatment and prognosis.

However, the approach adopted in this book has its limitation in the amount of detail that can be provided and it makes no allowances for controversial opinions.

This publication will be valuable to postgraduate doctors preparing for the MRCP and MRCS examinations, general practitioners, oncology nurses and basic science researchers in the field of oncology. It will also serve as a quick reference guide to medical and surgical oncologists.

I have made every effort to ensure that the information contained in this book is accurate at the date of going to press.

*London, 1998*                                                      KMM

# Common Abbreviations

| | |
|---|---|
| ACTH | adrenocorticotrophic hormone |
| ADH | antidiuretic hormone |
| AIDS | acquired immunodeficiency syndrome |
| BPH | benign prostatic hyperplasia |
| CSF | cerebrospinal fluid |
| CT | computed tomography |
| CXR | chest X-ray |
| DNA | deoxynucleic acid |
| ER | estrogen receptor |
| ERCP | endoscopic retrograde cholangiopancreatography |
| ESR | erythrocyte sedimentation rate |
| EUA | examination under anaesthetic |
| FBC | full blood count |
| FIGO | International Federation of Gynaecology and Obstetrics |
| FNAC | fine needle aspiration cytology |
| 5-FU | 5-fluorouracil |
| GI | gastrointestinal |
| HIV | human immunodeficiency virus |
| IVU | intravenous urogram |
| LFTs | liver function tests |
| [$^{125}$I]-MIBG | metiodobenzylguanidine |
| MEN | multiple endocrine neoplasia |
| MRI | magnetic resonance imaging |
| MTC | medullary thyroid cancer |
| MTH | medullary thyroid hyperplasia |
| OCP | oral contraceptive pill |
| PSA | prostatic specific antigen |
| PTH | parathyroid hormone |
| PTC | percutaneous transhepatic cholangiogram |
| PUVA | psoralen with ultraviolet radiation A (long wave) |
| SCC | squamous cell carcinoma |
| TNM | tumour/node/metastasis staging |
| TSH | thyroid stimulating hormone |
| TURP | transurethral prostatectomy |
| U&Es | urea and electrolytes |
| USS | ultrasound scan |
| UV | ultraviolet |
| VMA | vanilyl mandelic acid |

# 1. Oncogenesis

## Basic Principles

- Carcinogenesis is multistage.
- Initiation → Promotion → Cancer.
- Initiation is irreversible whereas promotion is reversible.
- Effects of initiation are inheritable.
- DNA structural changes lead to tumour development.

## Host Factors in Carcinogenesis

- Immune system.
- Endogenous hormones.
- Genetic factors such as oncogenes and tumour suppressor genes.

## Environmental Factors

- Radiation can cause DNA damage:
  - Ionising radiation includes X- and γ-rays and α- and β-particles.
  - Non-ionising radiation, e.g. UV light.
- Chemical carcinogens include:
  - Polycyclic hydrocarbons.
  - Aromatic amines.
  - Alkylating agents.
  - Blue asbestos.
  - Aflatoxin (hepatocellular carcinoma).

## Viruses

- Epstein–Barr virus (EBV). This is a DNA oncogenic virus. It is a member of the herpes virus family. It is associated with Burkitt's lymphoma and nasopharyngeal carcinoma.
- Hepatitis B virus (HBV). The incidence of hepatocellular carcinoma is increased by 200-fold in chronic carriers of HBV.
- Human papilloma virus (HPV). This virus is associated with cervical cancer and epidermodysplasia verruciformis (multiple squamous cell carcinomas of the skin).

- Human T-cell leukaemia virus (HTLV-1). This is an RNA virus. It is associated with several malignancies including leukaemias and lymphomas.

## Oncogenes

- Oncogenes are genes capable of causing malignancy. The normal gene is called a proto-oncogene.
- Methods of activation of oncogenes include:
  - Chromosomal rearrangements.
  - Point mutation.
  - Growth factors.

## Anti-oncogenes (Tumour-suppressor Genes)

- These are genes capable of suppressing neoplasia. Loss of these genes can result in neoplasia. Examples include p53 and retinoblastoma (RB1) genes.

# 2. Growth and Metastases

- Tumour cells can successfully metastasise if they have the ability to:
  - Regulate the production of proteases (by the tumour cells or surrounding stroma cells).
  - Regulate the production of adhesion molecules.
  - Regulate the expression of major histocompatibility complex (MHC) units and escape immune surveillance including natural killer cells.
  - Regulate the process of clotting.
  - Respond to cytokines and growth factors.

## The Metalloproteinases

- There are at least eight members of these lytic enzymes that are responsible for the degradation of the extracellular matrix (ECM).
- They are secreted by the stromal elements or the tumour cells.

## Cadherins

- These are transmembrane glycoproteins which mediate haemophilic adhesions between cells.
- Down-regulation of E-cadherins is associated with dedifferentiation and metastasis of cells.

## Integrins

- These are transmembrane proteins which mediate cell adhesion to the ECM proteins and transmit signals.

## The Sequential Steps of Metastasis

These include:
- Malignant transformation.
- Cell proliferation resulting in a primary tumour mass.
- Angiogenesis occurs when primary tumour exceeds 2 mm.
- Detachment of cells from primary tumour in association with down-regulation of E-cadherins.

- Detached tumour cells interact with ECM by integrins.
- Motility of tumour cells is stimulated by scatter factor secreted by fibroblasts or by motility factors secreted by the tumour cells.
- Metalloproteinases secreted by tumour cells or stromal fibroblasts degrade ECM and allow invasion of blood vessels and lymphatics.
- Within blood vessels/lymphatics some tumour cells are attacked by T-cells, others escape immune surveillance due to lack or altered major MHC units.
- Tumour cells adhere to endothelial cells via integrins, intracellular adhesion molecules, selectins, CD44 and other adhesion molecules.
- Tumour cell invasion of target tissues is facilitated by metalloproteinases which degrade ECM.

# 3. Principles of Chemotherapy

**The Cell Cycle**

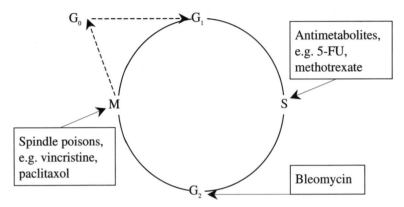

**Figure 1    The cell cycle. M = mitosis phase, $G_1$ = gap 1, S = synthesis phase, $G_2$ = gap 2 and $G_0$ = resting phase**

- The duration of the cell cycle is approximately 48 hours.
- Stimulatory signals come from cyclins (cyclins D and E in the $G_1$ phase, cyclin A in the S phase and cyclin B in the $G_2$ and M phases). Inhibitory signals come from tumour suppressor genes (e.g. p53 and RB1).
- Cytotoxic drugs kill tumour and normal cells, but tumour cells have a greater sensitivity to these drugs or a reduced ability to repair cytotoxic damage.
- Chemotherapy agents can be cycle specific, e.g. alkylating and inter-calating, or phase specific, e.g. spindle poisons and antimetabolites.

**Classification of Cytotoxic Drugs**

- Alkylating agents:
  - Chemically react with the structure forming methyl cross-bridges between the two strands of DNA base pairs. This prevents the DNA strands from coming apart during mitosis, and division therefore fails.
  - Examples include nitrogen mustards, melphalan, chorambucil, cyclophosphamide, busulphan, nitrosoureas, platinum and decarb-azine.
- Antimetabolites:
  - Inhibit the formation of essential nucleic acids thus interfering with

DNA/RNA synthesis and causing cell death.
- Examples include: methotrexate, 5-fluorouracil (5-FU), cytosine, arabinoside and purine analogues.
- Folinic acids can be given to rescue cells from the effect of methotrexate.
- Anti-tumour antibiotics:
  - Anthracyclines include doxorubicin, daunorubicin and epirubicin. These drugs intercalate between base pairs of DNA causing DNA damage. Mitoxantrone is structurally related to this group of drugs.
  - Bleomycin. This drug is $G_2$ specific.
  - Mitomycin C acts as an alkylating agent and generates free radicals capable of causing DNA damage.
  - Actinomycin D intercalates between guanine and cytosine thus inhibiting DNA/RNA synthesis.
  - Platinum analogues (cisplatin and carboplatin).
- Plant-derived cytotoxic drugs:
  - Vinca alkaloids. Vincristine, vinblastine and vindesine inhibit the formation of mitotic spindles by binding to tubulin.
  - Epidophyllotoxins, e.g. etoposide. These drugs interfere with topoisomerase II enzymes causing DNA damage during the S phase.
  - Paclitaxol inhibits mitosis by promoting a disorganised and stabilised assembly of microtubules. It is a new drug and mainly used in the treatment of breast and ovarian cancers.
- Other drugs:
  - Decarbazine is an alkylating agent used in the treatment of melanoma.
  - Procarbazine is used to treat Hodgkin's lymphoma.

## Chemotherapy Protocols

- Combinations are usually used.
- Pulsed or intermittent therapy is frequently used in order to allow a larger dose to be given.
- High-dose chemotherapy can be given with the use of haematopoietic growth factors, stem cell support or autologous bone marrow transplantation in order to encounter myelosuppression.

## Mechanisms of Drug Resistance

- Increased concentrations of target enzymes, e.g. doxorubicin, epirubicin, paclitaxol, vincristine, etc.
- Reduced uptake by tumour cells, e.g. daunorubicin.

- Increased activity of salvage pathways, e.g. antimetabolites.
- Detoxification.
- Improved DNA repair mechanisms by target cells.
- Impairment of activation or increased inactivation of the drug.

# 4. Principles of Radiotherapy

## Basic Principles

- The commonest type of ionising radiation used in clinical practice is X-rays which are produced artificially by accelerating electrons (linear accelerators) using microwave energy, resulting in therapeutic megavolt beams.
- Gamma rays are identical to X-rays but arise from the decay of radioactive isotopes.
- Ionising radiation causes irreversible DNA damage directly or indirectly by generating toxic free radicals. The DNA damage, which is oxygen dependent, is the most important factor in cell killing.
- Radiotherapy dose is expressed in grays or centigrays ($1\,Gy = 100\,cGy$) and describes the energy absorbed per unit mass of tissue.
- Fractionation allows a higher degree of radiation to be given.

## Clinical Applications

- Cancer patients are treated by external beam radiation (linear accelerator or cobalt machine) or insertion of a radioactive material in body tissues (interstitial radiotherapy) or cavities (intracavity radiotherapy).
- Radiotherapy can be palliative or curative. It can be combined with other treatment modalities such as surgery and chemotherapy. Pre-operative radiotherapy may be given in order to render a tumour operable. Post-operative radiotherapy is used mainly to reduce the rate of local recurrence.
- The effects of radiotherapy depend on the dose, the tumour size, the tumour proliferation rate, hypoxia, tumour radiosensitivity, patient's performance, the presence of anaemia and vascular disease.

## Side Effects

- Early side effects include mucositis, alopecia, skin erythema, nausea, vomiting, enteritis and bone marrow suppression. These side effects are reversible and can be managed symptomatically.
- Late side effects include spinal cord myelitis, pneumonitis, strictures, telangiectasia and secondary cancers. Approximately 3% of patients develop a second cancer 15 years after treatment.

# 5. Cancer of the Lip

**Epidemiology**

- The incidence is higher among Caucasians (versus blacks), smokers and outdoor workers.

**Pathology**

- Smoking (especially pipe smoking) and solar radiation are important aetiological factors.
- Squamous cell carcinoma (SCC) is the commonest histological type. Basal cell carcinoma is occasionally seen.
- 92% of lesions occur on the lower lip, 5% occur on the upper lip and 3% at the angle of the mouth.
- Submandibular nodes are the usual sites for metastases.

**Investigation**

- Limited surgical biopsy under local anaesthetic.
- Fine needle aspriration cytology (FNAC) of enlarged lymph nodes.

**Treatment**

- Surgery and radiotherapy are equally effective.
- Surgical defects following adequate excision can be reconstructed using local flaps (from the opposite lip) or closed primarily if small.
- The cure rate is 90%.

# 6. Oral Cancer

## Epidemiology

- It accounts for 4% of all cancers (India has the highest incidence).
- Peak incidence 50–70 years.
- Commoner in men.

## Pathology

- Squamous cell carcinoma (SCC) accounts for 90% of all cases.
- Adenocarcinoma accounts for 3% of cases.
- Kaposi's sarcoma, lymphoma and melanoma are rare.

## Aetiology

Risk factors include:

- Smoking.
- Alcohol.
- Infections (syphilis, candidiasis and herpes virus).
- Immunosuppression.
- Industrial hazards (textile workers).
- Oncogenes (ras, p53, L-myc and C-myc).
- Leukoplakia.
- Erythroplakia.

## Clinical Presentation

- Ulcerating lesions.
- Exophytic lesions.
- Induration.
- Swelling.
- Pain.
- Pathological mandibular fractures.
- Paraesthesia along the inferior alveolar nerve distribution.
- Lymphadenopathy in the head and neck region.

## Investigations

- Exfoliative cytology.
- Surgical biopsy including a margin of healthy tissue.
- CT and MRI.
- FNAC of enlarged lymph nodes.
- Plain radiograph of adjacent teeth may be useful.

## Treatment

- SCC of the anterior two thirds of the tongue:
    - This can be treated with surgical excision (with a 1 mm margin) or radiotherapy.
    - Large surgical defects can be reconstructed using split thickness skin grafts, local skin flaps (forehead or deltopectoral), myocutaneous flaps (pectoralis major or trapezius) or free flaps (microvascular anastomosis).
- SCC in the floor of the mouth:
    - If the alveolar process is involved then wide local excision with reconstruction (local or free flaps) is appropriate.
    - If the alveolar process is not involved, then radiotherapy is the treatment of choice.
- SCC on the mandibular alveolus is treated with surgical excision and reconstruction using bone grafting or a free flap using the underlying bone (radial forearm flap)
- SCC of the buccal mucosa is treated with surgical resection and the defect is reconstructed with local or free flap
- SCC on the upper jaw is treated with surgical excision and reconstruction using a prosthetic appliance lined with skin graft is necessary.

# 7. Salivary Glands

## Epidemiology

- Incidence is 1.5 per 100 000 per year.
- 70% of the lesions occur in the parotid (20% are malignant).

## Aetiology

- Malignant transformation of a pleomorphic adenoma.
- Radiation.
- Association with breast cancer.

## Pathology

- The grade (high grade and low grade) is more important than the histological type (acinic cell, mucoepidermoid and carcinoma) in predicting behaviour and prognosis.

## Clinical Presentation

- Swelling (rate of growth depends upon grade of tumour).
- Facial nerve palsy (parotid tumours).
- Sensory loss of anterior two thirds of tongue (submandibular tumours).
- Trismus and pain along trigeminal nerve distribution.
- Lymphadenopathy (25% of cases).

## Investigations

- Core biopsy is more reliable than FNAC.
- Open biopsy.
- CT or MRI.
- Staging investigations includes CXR, thoracic CT and bone scan.

**Management**

- Surgical excision for low grade tumours.
- Surgical excision followed by radiotherapy for high grade tumours.
- The facial nerve may be sacrificed in some cases.
- Neck dissection is indicated in the presence of lymph node metastases (confirmed by FNAC).
- Pre-operative radiotherapy followed by surgery for locally advanced tumours.
- Radiotherapy alone has a local control rate of 30% in patients with locally advanced tumours.
- Plastic reconstruction may be performed using pectoralis major, trapezius and latissimus dorsi myocutaneous flaps or radial forearm free flap.

**Prognosis**

- Low-grade tumours: the 10-year survival rate is 90%.
- High-grade tumour: the 10-year survival rate is 25%.

# 8. Retinoblastoma

## Epidemiology

- The incidence is 1 per 15 000 live births.
- It accounts for 3% of all childhood malignancies.
- The incidence is increasing. It has doubled in the last 40 years.

## Aetiology

- Most cases are sporadic.
- Some cases are inherited in an autosomal dominant fashion. Sporadic bilateral retinoblastoma and familial retinoblastoma are inheritable.
- The retinoblastoma (Rb) gene is a growth suppressor gene. Its product has a general suppressive function in the cell cycle.

## Pathology

- The tumour usually consists of undifferentiated and small cells with deeply staining nuclei and scanty cytoplasm.
- The tumour is usually multifocal.
- The commonest mode of metastases is via the blood stream to bone marrow, liver, lungs and lymph nodes.

## Clinical Features

- The tumour usually presents before the age of 2 years.
- 'White pupil' is the commonest presentation.
- Other features include strabismus, glaucoma, defect in visual fixation and inflammatory changes within the eye.
- Ophthalmological assessment is required in such cases. Surgical biopsy is not recommended.

## Investigations

- Full blood count (FBC), bone scan, CXR.
- Orbital CT or MRI.

• Analysis of CSF if intracranial spread is suspected.

## Management

• Cryosurgery or photocoagulation for very small lesions.
• Brachytherapy (for lesions measuring 3–10 mm) using radioactive cobalt.
• External beam radiation (35–40 Gy in 4 weeks) for large lesions and for lesions near the optic disc and macula.
• Eye enucleation for tumours unresponsive to conservative management and for tumour infiltrating the optic nerve. Post-operative radiotherapy may be given in such cases.
• Chemotherapy may be used for extraocular disease. Effective agents include vincristine, actinomycin D, doxorubicin, methotrexate and cyclophosphamide.
• Genetic counselling is an important part of management.

## Prognosis

• The cure rate for stages I and II is 100%.
• The cure rate for stages IV and V is 75%.
• The overall mortality is 10%.

# 9. Laryngeal Cancer

## Epidemiology

- Laryngeal cancer accounts for 2–3% of all malignant disease.
- The male to female ratio is 10:1.
- The disease occurs exclusively in smokers.
- The peak age of onset is 60 years.

## Pathology

- Squamous cell carcinoma accounts for most cases.
- Adenoid cystic carcinoma and sarcoma are rare.
- Laryngeal cancer can be classified into four types according to site or origin:
  - Glottic (60%).
  - Supraglottic (30%).
  - Subglottic (5%).
  - Marginal (5%).
- The disease spread is local initially.
- Lymphatic spread to deep cervical lymph nodes.
- Pulmonary metastases are occasionally seen.

## Clinical Features

- Hoarseness is the main symptom of the disease.
- Other symptoms include:
  - Dysphagia.
  - Ear ache.
  - Dyspnoea.
  - Haemoptysis.

## Investigations

- Microlaryngoscopy and biopsy.
- CXR.
- CT to define the extent of the disease.

**Treatment**

- Glottic tumours:
  - Carcinoma *in situ* can be treated with local excision of involved mucosa. T1 and T2 lesions are effectively treated with radiotherapy. The resulting voice quality is better than after partial (vertical) laryngectomy. Salvage surgery in the form of partial or total laryngectomy is performed where failure occurs with radiotherapy treatment.
  - Tumours involving the contralateral cord and/or regional lymph nodes can be treated with total laryngectomy combined with neck dissection. Post-operative radiotherapy may be given.
- Early supraglottic tumours are treated by preoperative radiotherapy and subsequent total laryngectomy.
- Advanced supraglottic, subglottic and glottic tumours are treated with radiotherapy, chemotherapy and/or surgery.
- Following total laryngectomy, 60% of patients develop a reasonable oesophageal speech. Many patients are now provided with a valve fitted to a tracheopharyngeal fistula. Phonation is produced by occluding the tracheostomy with a finger.
- Tracheostomy care training, speech therapy and social support are important aspects of management.

**Prognosis**

- The cure rate for T1 and T2 lesions is 90% and 65%, respectively.
- The 5-year survival for T3 tumours is 25%.

# 10. Lung Cancer

## Epidemiology

- It is the most common form of cancer in Western countries.
- The male to female ratio is 4:1.

## Aetiology

- Prolonged exposure to cigarette smoke is the most important aetiological factor.
- Asbestos exposure.
- Industrial pollution, e.g. coal and tar fumes, nickel, zinc, etc.
- Occupational exposure to nickel, chromium, iron oxide and arsenicals.

## Pathology

- Squamous cell carcinoma (40%) tends to arise proximally in large bronchi. It is associated with loss of heterozygosity of the p53 gene.
- Small cell lung cancer (20%). Neurosecretory granules are often present and produce various hormones such as calcitonin, ADH, ACTH, PTH, etc. It is associated with over-expression of C-myc and loss of heterozygosity of p53.
- Adenocarcinoma (15–50%) tends to arise in scars and peripheral sites. It is more common in females. It may be bronchoalveolar or broncho-acinar. It is less related to smoking than the other types.
- Large cell carcinoma (10%).
- Mixed histologies (15%).
- Carcinoid tumours (< 1%).
- Sarcoma (< 1%).

Carcinoma of the bronchus spreads by local invasion and by lymphatic and haematogenous routes.

## Clinical Features

- The commonest symptoms are haemoptysis, cough, dyspnoea and chest pain.

- Other features include:
  - Hoarseness.
  - Pleural effusion.
  - Phrenic nerve palsy.
  - Pneumonia.
  - Pulmonary collapse.
  - Dysphagia.
  - Stridor.
  - Superior vena cava obstruction (SVCO).
  - Pancoast tumour.
  - Mass in the neck.
  - Bone metastases.
  - Anorexia.
  - Weight loss.
  - Hypercalcaemia.
  - SIADH (syndrome of inappropriate ADH secretion).
  - Cushing's syndrome.
  - Features of metastases to brain and intraperitoneal cavity.

**Investigations**

- CXR.
- Exfoliative sputum cytology (four specimens).
- Brochoscopy and biopsy.
- CT scanning to define tumour extent.
- Mediastinoscopy to assess extent of disease.
- Other investigations include:
  - FBC.
  - Serum biochemistry.
  - Bone scan.
  - Liver USS.
  - Brain CT.
  - Lymph node biopsy.
  - Pleural fluid cytology, etc.

**Staging (TNM System)**

- Stage I:   $T_{1,2}, N_0, M_0$
             $T_1, N_1, M_0$
- Stage II:  $T_2, N_1, M_0$
- Stage III: Any $T_3$

Any N$_2$
Any M$_1$

## Treatment and Prognosis

- Non-small cell lung cancer (NSCLC):
  - Less than 50% of cases are resectable at the time of diagnosis.
  - Operable cases may be treated by wedge excision (for localised peripheral tumours), lobectomy (for more centrally located tumours), or pneumectomy (for tumours of the main bronchus where more than one lobe is involved or the hilum is involved).
  - The 5-year survival for resectable tumours is 55% for stage I, 30% for stage II and 18% for stage III. T$_1$ squamous cell tumours have the best survival rate (80%).
  - Radical radiotherapy (60 Gy over 6 weeks) is indicated in patients with resectable tumours but who are unfit for surgery or refuse surgery. The 5-year survival is 10%.
  - Palliative radiotherapy to relieve troublesome symptoms in patients with inoperable disease.
  - Chemotherapy has a limited role in localised NSCLC. The benefit is estimated to be 5%. Drugs used include mitomycin, cisplatin, cyclophosphamide, doxorubicin, etc. The drugs may be given in combination before or after radiotherapy or surgery.
- Small cell lung cancer (SCLC):
  - The majority of patients present with extensive disease.
  - Radiotherapy is the mainstay of treatment for locoregional disease and metastases. The primary tumour response rate is 80% with 50 Gy over 5 weeks.
  - Combination chemotherapy (doxorubicin, etoposide and cyclophosphamide) is indicated in fit patients.
  - The 2-year survival rate for limited disease is 15%.

## Gene Therapy

- Introduction of the wild type p53 plus a viral vector (e.g. an adenovirus) into advanced pulmonary tumours is being currently investigated. The initial results are encouraging.

# 11.  Breast Cancer

## Epidemiology

- Breast cancer is the leading cause of death among women.
- The lifetime risk is approximately 9%.
- The average incidence is 65 per $10^5$ persons per year.

## Aetiology

- The risk factors include:
  - Early menarche (the relative risk is 1.5).
  - Late menopause (early menopause is protective).
  - Obesity after the menopause (pre-menopausal obesity is protective).
  - Null parity increases risk by 30%.
  - Pregnancy after the age of 35.
  - Benign breast disease, especially atypical epithelial hyperplasia.
  - Oral contraceptives.
  - Hormone replacement therapy seems to increase the risk by 75% after use for 6 years.
  - Family history of breast cancer. The risk is particularly high in the first degree relatives of patients with early onset of breast cancer (< 45 years) and/or bilateral breast cancer.
  - Diet – it is thought that red meat and fat increase the risk. High-fibre diet and antioxidant vitamins may have a protective effect.
  - Alcohol. Consumption is associated with increased risk.
  - Ionising radiation. The risk increases with radiation dose. Exposure during the second decade has a maximal risk. The latency period is 15–20 years.

## Screening

- Screening mammography is recommended for:
  - All women aged 50–65 years (every 2 years).
  - All women with a previous history of breast cancer or a significant family history of breast cancer.
- Screening mammography has been shown to reduce breast cancer mortality by 30% in women aged over 50 years.
- All women are advised to perform self examination on a monthly basis.

**Pathology**

- Ductal carcinoma *in situ* (DCIS) is confined to the duct-lobular units without breaching the basement membrane. It is subclassified into
  - Comedo DCIS (high nuclear grade, HNG).
  - Solid DCIS (usually HNG).
  - Cribriform (usually low nuclear grade, LNG).
  - Micropapillary (usually LNG).
  - Intracystic papillary.
  - Endocrine.
  - Cystic hypersecretory.

  The risk of developing into invasive cancer is approximately 50%.
- Lobular carcinoma *in situ* (LCIS). This is a tumour marker. The risk of developing invasive cancer is 25% after 20 years. The invasive lesion may be ductal.
- Infiltrating ductal carcinoma. This is the commonest type.
- Infiltrating lobular carcinoma. This type is associated with a higher incidence of bilateral breast cancer.
- Colloid carcinoma:
  - It accounts for 5% of breast cancers.
  - It has a good prognosis.
- Tubular carcinoma has an excellent prognosis.
- Cribriform carcinoma is rare and has a good prognosis.
- Papillary carcinoma is rare and has a good prognosis.
- Medullary carcinoma has a good prognosis.
- Paget's disease of the breast. There is skin infiltration by large pale staining cells.
- Inflammatory carcinoma accounts for 2% of all cases. There is erythema, tenderness and invasion of the dermal lymphatics by tumour cells.
- Squamous cell carcinoma:
  - This is a rare tumour.
  - The prognosis is similar to that of infiltrating ductal cell carcinoma.
  - A primary extra-mammary lesion should be excluded.

**Clinical Features**

- Symptoms include:
  - Breast lump (85%).
  - Pain (5%).
  - Nipple retraction (5%).
  - Nipple discharge (2%).

- Paget's disease (5%).
- Axillary mass (1%).
- Skin changes (1%).
- Distant metastases.
- Clinical examination usually reveals a solid mass which may be ill-defined and fixed to overlying/underlying structures.
- The locoregional lymph nodes, thoracic spine and abdomen should be examined in the search for metastases.
- Breast cancer may present as an impalpable mammographic abnormality during screening. DCIS accounts for 20% of screen-detected cancers.

**Investigations**

- FNAC:
  - It has a high specificity (> 98%) in the hands of experienced cytologists.
  - It cannot distinguish between infiltrating and *in situ* lesions.
  - Can be performed stereotactically for impalpable lesions.
- Core biopsy:
  - It has a lower sensitivity than FNAC.
  - It is indicated if neoadjuvant chemotherapy is considered, if mastectomy is planned and for impalpable lesions (under stereotactic guidance).
- Mammography:
  - Signs of malignancy, including spiculated masses, circumscribed masses, microcalcification, stellate lesions, parenchymal distortions, skin tethering and retraction, and nipple inversion.
- Ultrasound examination (± Doppler).
- Cytological analysis of scrape smear (of nipple) and nipple discharge.
- MRI of the breast (role is still being defined).
- Investigations for suspected metastatic disease including:
  - FBC, serum biochemistry and CXR (all patients).
  - Liver USS and bone scan for patients with stage II, III and IV disease.
  - Bone MRI has been recently used with success.

**Management**

- Localised breast cancer:
  - This is treated by a wide local excision (with a minimal clear margin of 2 cm) combined with axillary dissection (Level I, II and III) and followed by radiotherapy to the whole breast. Axillary dissection is

not necessary for *in situ* cancer as the incidence of node metastases is
< 1%.

- The wider the clear margin, the lower the local recurrence rate.
- The indications for mastectomy include a large carcinoma (> 4 cm), multifocal disease, recurrent disease, centrally located tumour, DCIS component > 40 mm and the patient's request to have a mastectomy.
- All patients with ER-positive invasive breast cancer should receive tamoxifen (20 mg daily) for 5 years. The benefit of tamoxifen therapy is significantly reduced in patients with ER-negative tumours.
- Fit patients with poor prognosis factors such as positive nodes, grade III tumours, ER negative and lymphovascular invasion, should receive systemic chemotherapy, e.g. cyclophosphamide, methotrexate and 5-FU (CMF); 6 courses are usually given.
- In patients with extensive nodal involvement, a high-dose chemotherapy with autogenous stem-cell support is considered.
- Radiotherapy to the axilla is indicated for extracapsular axillary spread.
- Radiotherapy to the breast may be omitted for good prognosis tumours, e.g. < 1 cm, tubular papillary and mucoid carcinoma.
- Systemic adjuvant therapy (including tamoxifen and cytotoxic chemotherapy) reduces mortality by 20–30% at 10 years.
- Pre-operative neoadjuvant chemotherapy may permit conservation surgery for large breast cancers. However, this approach does not seem to prolong survival.
- Paget's disease of the breast is treated by simple mastectomy (no palpable breast tumour) or Patey's mastectomy (palpable breast tumour). Pure Paget's disease may be treated by a local excision and radiotherapy, thus conserving the breast.

- Locally advanced breast cancer (LABC):
  - LABC is initially treated by chemotherapy (e.g. doxorubicin), tamoxifen and/or aromatase inhibitors, followed by surgical excision (mastectomy or wide local excision) or radical radiotherapy (if the tumour is inoperable). The dose of radical radiotherapy is 65–80 Gy. Systemic therapy will be continued after surgery/radiotherapy.
- Metastatic breast cancer:
  - Pre-menopausal patients are treated by a combination chemotherapy and/or hormonal therapy such as LHRH agonists and tamoxifen. Chemotherapeutic regimens include CMF, EFC (epirubicin, 5-FU and cyclophosphamide), MMM (mitozantrone, methotrexate and mitomycin) and Taxol. The response rate is 50%.
  - Post-menopausal patients are primarily treated by tamoxifen followed by aromatase inhibitors such as anastrozole.
  - Radiotherapy for bone and CNS metastases.

- Other endocrine agents include progestogens and aminoglutethimide.
- Other management modalities include Le-Veen shunt for ascites, pleurodesis (tetracycline, bleomycin or talc) for recurrent effusions, analgesia, correction of hypercalcaemia, surgical fixation of fractures, bisphonates such as clodronate (for bony metastases) and psychological support.
- Breast reconstruction:
  - Methods available include implant reconstruction, expandable prosthesis, latissimus dorsi flap and transverse rectus abdominis myocutaneous flap (pedicled or free).
  - Nipple areola reconstruction, using a full-thickness skin graft from the groin or contralateral nipple, can be performed.
  - Breast reconstruction can be performed at the time of mastectomy without compromising oncological outcome.
- The specialist breast cancer nurse plays an important role in management.

## Prognosis

- Axillary node status is the best single predictor of prognosis.
- Other prognostic parameters include tumour size, tumour grade, ER status and lymphovascular invasion.
- The 10-year survival rate for node-negative patients is 72% versus 35% for node-positive patients.
- 99% of DCIS lesions are cured by mastectomy.

## Follow-Up

- Six-monthly review for breast conservation surgery patients and yearly review for mastectomy patients.
- Annual mammography.
- During follow up, one should remember that lobular carcinoma tends to metastasise to the GI tract.

## Familial Breast Cancer

- This accounts for 5% of all breast cancers.
- Genes responsible include the BRCA-1 gene on 17q21, the BRCA-2 gene on 13q12–13 (uncloned), the p53 gene on 17p13, the ataxia telangectasia gene on 11q23 and the androgen receptor gene on the X-chromosome.

**Recent Advances**

- It is likely that the sentinel node biopsy through a 2 cm incision will replace routine axillary node dissection. If the sentinel node contains metastatic disease, then axillary clearance is performed. The sentinel node can be accurately localised using planar scintigraphy and intra-operative gamma probe.
- Postmastectomy radiotherapy has been shown to reduce logical recurrence and mortality in premenopausal women with node-positive disease who have received chemotherapy. Similar results are expected for postmenopausal women.
- There is increasing evidence that screening during the fifth decade (40–49 years) may be effective.

# 12.  Oesophagus

## Epidemiology

- The incidence varies from 3 to 180 per 100 000 per year depending upon geographical location.
- There is a geographic clustering in certain parts of Asia and Africa.
- The male to female ratio is 7.

## Aetiology

The risk factors include:
- Barrett's oesophagus (risk 13%).
- Achalasia.
- Corrosive strictures.
- Diverticular disease of the oesophagus.
- Plummer–Vinson syndrome.
- Other risk factors include smoking, alcohol, vitamin C deficiency, zinc deficiency and tylosis.

## Pathology

- In Asia, 80% of carcinomas are of squamous cell type and 15% are adenocarcinoma. The middle third is the commonest location.
- In Western countries, 45% are adenocarcinomas and 50% are squamous cell carcinomas. Lesions of the lower oesophagus and cardia are more common in these countries.

## Clinical Presentation

- Dysphagia (95%).
- Regurgitation (45%).
- Weight loss (40%).
- Cough (25%).
- Pain (20%).
- Hoarse voice (20%).
- Dyspnoea (5%).
- Haemoptysis (5%).

- Haematemesis (5%).
- Neck mass (5%).
- Anaemia.


**Physical Examination**

- Search for metastases in the neck (Virchow's node), abdomen and pelvis.


**Investigations**

- Double contrast barium swallow.
- Upper GI endoscopy (biopsy or brush cytology).
- Endoscopic ultrasound (most precise staging investigation).
- CT or MRI of thorax and abdomen.
- Other investigations include:
  - FBC.
  - Liver function tests (LFTs).
  - CXR.
  - Bronchoscopy.
  - Abdominal USS.


**Treatment**

- Oesophageal resection:
  - This is indicated for operable tumours (40% of all cases).
  - It requires perioperative intensive care facilities and patient's fitness.
  - A proximal margin of 10 cm is preferable.
  - It should be combined with removal of regional lymph nodes in juxta position.
  - The Ivor–Lewis operation is suitable for tumours of the middle and lower thirds. The operation usually requires a laparotomy and a thoracotomy. The stomach is pulled through for anastomosis with the proximal oesophagus and a pyloroplasty is performed.
  - For tumours of the upper third, McKeown's procedure (laparotomy, right thoracotomy and left neck incision) or a sternotomy approach are used. A stomach pull-through or a jejunal Roux-en-Y can be performed. In some cases, laryngectomy, tracheostomy, pharyngectomy and/or total oesophagectomy may be required.
  - Thoracoscopic dissection of the oesophagus has been recently

developed.
  • Surgery also has a palliative role (surgical bypass).
• Radiotherapy:
  • The response rate is 35%.
  • The complete eradication rate is 5%.
  • Side effects include strictures, cardiac and pulmonary damage, bleeding and malignant oesophago-tracheo-bronchial fistula formation.
• Intubation:
  • For advanced and non-resectable tumours and for unfit patients.
  • Pulsion or traction technique may be used.
  • The funnel of the tube sits proximal to the tumour.
  • Self-expanding metal stents have been used recently with good results.
  • The risk of perforation is 10%.
  • Intubation is contraindicated in cervical lesions.
• Laser therapy:
  • Nd:YAG laser provides temporary palliation.
  • Temporary palliation.
• Chemotherapy
  • There is increasing evidence that chemotherapy (e.g. 5-FU and cisplatin) is effective in oesophageal cancer. Tumour regression occurs in 60% of cases.

**Prognosis**

• The five-year suvival rate is 4% for surgery and 6% for radiography.

# 13.  Gastric Cancer

## Epidemiology

- The incidence is 23 per 100 000 per year (declining world-wide).
- It accounts for 6% of all cancer deaths.
- The peak incidence 50–70 years.
- The male to female ratio is 2.
- The highest incidence is in Japan.
- Premalignant changes include chronic atrophic gastritis, intestinal metaplasia and dysplasia. Risk factors include *Helicobacter pylori* infection, blood group A, high intake of salt and salt cured meats, vitamin deficiency (A, C and E) and high intake of nitrates.
- Various genetic alterations have been linked to gastric cancer, e.g. p53, C-myc and C-erb B2.

## Pathology

- The lesion may be polypoid, ulcerative, diffuse or ulcerative/diffuse.
- 35% of lesions arise in the proximal third.

## Clinical Features

- Dysphagia.
- Vomiting.
- Abdominal pain (50%).
- Epigastric mass (20%).
- Microcytic anaemia.
- Weight loss and cachexia.
- Other features include:
  - Krukenberg's tumour.
  - Venous thrombosis.
  - Left supraclavicular lymphadenopathy.

## Investigations

- FBC, serum biochemistry.
- Upper GI endoscopy (and biopsy) and barium meal.
- CT or MRI and/or USS for staging.

**Treatment**

- Gastrectomy:
  - Possible in 65% of cases.
  - Access through a transverse subcostal incision, vertical midline incision or Ivor–Lewis approach.
  - The omentum is removed in all cases.
  - Radically is classified into R1, R2 and R3 depending upon the level of lymph node dissection.
  - For proximal tumours – oesophageal resection may be required to achieve a 10 cm proximal margin.
  - Billroth II reconstruction for distal tumours.
  - Radical total gastrectomy and oesophago-jejunostomy (Roux-en-Y) for extensive tumours.
- Radiotherapy may be given pre-, intra- or postoperatively.
- Chemotherapy. 5-FU, mitomycin C and adriamycin may be given in advanced disease.
- Palliative procedures include gastroenterostomy (ante-colic), intubation, dilatation and laser treatment.

**Prognosis**

- The 5-year survival is 40% (Japanese series).
- In Western series, the 5-year survival is 20%.

# 14. Gastrointestinal Lymphoma (GIL)

**Epidemiology**

- GIL represents 5% of all GI malignancies.
- It is essential to distinguish between primary GIL and secondary involvement of the GI tract.
- The peak incidence occurs during 50–70 years.
- The male to female ratio is 2:1.
- The incidence of anorectal lymphoma is rising.

**Aetiology**

- Malignant transformation of mucosa-associated lymphatic tissue (MALT) seems to be important in pathogenesis.
- The predisposing factors include:
  - Atrophic gastritis (*Helicobacter pylori*).
  - α-chain disease.
  - Coeliac disease.
  - Dermatitis herpatiformis.
  - Crohn's disease.
  - Auto immune disorders.
  - Immunodeficiency syndromes including AIDS.

**Pathology**

- Stage I:    Tumour confined to GI organs.
- Stage II:   Tumour with intra-abdominal lymph node involvement.
- Stage III:  Extra-abdominal nodes or other organs are involved.
- Stage IV:  Disseminated disease.

There are three main types:
- Western lymphoma (non-Hodgkin's B-cell lymphoma).
- Primary lymphoma associated with coeliac disease (T-cell lymphoma).
- Mediterranean lymphoma associated with α-chain disease.

## Clinical Features

- The symptoms include:
  - Abdominal pain.
  - Nausea.
  - Vomiting.
  - Weight loss.
  - Fatigue.
- Physical examination may reveal an abdominal mass (35%) and anaemia.
- Symptoms and signs of obstruction, perforation or haemorrhage.

## Investigations

- FBC, serum U&Es and LFTs.
- CXR (with thoracic CT).
- Abdominal ultrasonography.
- Abdomino-pelvic CT.
- Gastrointestinal endoscopy (with biopsy).
- Endosonography.
- Barium studies of the GI tract.
- Faecal occult blood testing.
- Southern blot DNA hybridisation of fresh biopsy specimens.
- Laparotomy/laparoscopy.

## Management

- Treatment depends upon the site, stage and histological subtype:
  - Stage I and II disease is treated by resection of the involved segment (e.g. subtotal gastrectomy, right hemicolectomy, etc.) with the regional lymph nodes. Post-operative radiotherapy (25 Gy to the whole abdomen with a boost of 15 Gy to the tumour region) and chemotherapy with cyclophosphamide, doxorubicin, vincristine and prednisolone (CHOP) are recommended if the lesion is high grade and/or the margins of the resection specimens are involved by the disease.
  - Stage III and IV disease is treated by chemotherapy (CHOP) and radiotherapy with 50% response rate. Surgical intervention is reserved for complications such as obstruction, haemorrhage and perforation.

**Prognosis**

- The 5-year survival rate for stages I and II is 70% for completely resected tumours and 40% for incompletely resected lesions.
- The 5-year survival for stages III and IV is 20%.

# 15. Small Bowel Carcinoma

**Epidemiology**

- It accounts for 40% of all small bowel malignancies. The latter accounts for 5% of all GI malignancies.
- It is twice as common in men as in women.
- The average age at presentation is 50 years.
- The duodenum and proximal jejunum are the commonest sites.

**Aetiology**

- The predisposing factors include Crohn's disease, coeliac disease, Peutz–Jegher's syndrome, adenomatous polyps and polyposis syndromes.

**Clinical Features**

- The symptoms are:
  - Diarrhoea.
  - Anaemia.
  - Abdominal pain.
  - Nausea.
  - Vomiting.
  - Haemorrhage.
  - Perforation.
  - Intermittent jaundice (duodenal lesions).
  - Anorexia.
  - Weight loss.
- The signs include:
  - Anaemia.
  - Abdominal mass.
  - Jaundice.
  - Signs of obstruction or perforation.

**Investigations**

- FBC, serum U&Es, LFTs, faecal occult blood testing.

- Barium meal and follow-through series reveal tumour in 50% of cases.
- GI endoscopy and biopsy.
- CXR.
- Abdominal USS and/or CT.
- Laparoscopy/laparotomy.

**Management**

- Wide surgical resection including the regional lymph nodes is the mainstay of management.
- Whipple's operation may be necessary for duodenal lesions.
- Surgical palliation may involve intestinal resection or bypass.
- Radiotherapy and chemotherapy play little role in the treatment.
- The role of nitrosoureas and 5-FU is currently being investigated.

**Prognosis**

- The lesions are usually advanced at the time of diagnosis.
- The incidence of metastases is approximately 70% at the time of laparotomy.
- The 5-year survival rate is 35% for duodenal lesions and 20% for lesions elsewhere.

*Note:*

Other primary malignancies of the small bowel include:
- Carcinoids (30%).
- Lymphoma (18%).
- Sarcoma (15%).

# 16. Colorectal Carcinoma

**Epidemiology**

- The incidence varies from 0.4 (Nigeria) per 100 000 per year to 32.3 (USA) per 100 000 per year.

**Aetiology**

- The risk factors include:
  - Familial polyposis coli (FAP).
  - Lynch syndrome I and II.
  - High intake of dietary fat.
  - Low intake of dietary fibre.
  - Obesity.
  - High alcohol intake.
  - Bile acids.
  - Tobacco smoking.
  - Asbestos.
  - Ulcerative colitis.
  - Crohn's disease.
  - Family history of colorectal cancer.
  - Previous history of colorectal polyps or cancer.
  - Ureterosigmoidostomy.
- The adenoma–carcinoma sequence is important in colorectal carcinogenesis.
- Genetic alterations in growth suppressor genes (p53 and BRCA-1) and oncogenes (K-ras) cause tissue change from normal epithelium to adenoma and then carcinoma.

**Screening**

- Patients with colorectal cancer, polyps, ulcerative colitis and family history of polyposis syndromes should be screened with colonoscopy.
- Other screening methods include flexible sigmoidoscopy and faecal occult blood (FOB) testing.

**Pathology**

- 98% of cancers are adenocarcinomas. The tumour is confined to the mucosal and sub-mucosal layers in Dukes A, has penetrated the bowel wall (muscularis mucosa) in Dukes B and there is regional lymph node involvement in Dukes C. There are distant metastases in Dukes D.
- The incidence of lymph node metastasis depends upon the tumour grade and the presence of p53 oncogenes.

**Clinical Features**

- Large bowel obstruction (more likely with left-sided lesions).
- Perforation and peritonitis.
- Altered bowel habits.
- Rectal bleeding.
- Microcytic anaemia (more likely with right-sided lesions).
- Small bowel obstruction (e.g. caecal carcinoma).
- Abdominal mass.
- Symptoms and signs of metastasis such as hepatomegaly and ascites.

**Investigations**

- Proctosigmoidoscopy.
- FBC.
- LFTs.
- Serum CEA (carcinoembryonic antigen).
- Barium enema.
- Colonoscopy.
- Abdominal ultrasonography (including liver).
- Endoscopic biopsy.
- Abdominopelvic CT.
- Other investigations include:
    - IVU for suspected ureter involvement.
    - Bone scan.
    - CXR and brain CT for suspected metastases.

**Treatment**

- Surgical excision is the main treatment. Right hemicolectomy, trans-verse colectomy, left hemicolectomy, sigmoid colectomy, anterior and

abdominoperineal excision of the rectum may be performed:
- The amount of large bowel removed depends upon the aetiology, arterial blood supply, and grade of differentiation, quality of anal sphincter and the patient's age and fitness
- A permanent stoma is necessary if the tumour invades the anal sphincters, the tumour is located within 5 cm of the dentate line and is poorly differentiated or the anal sphincters are weak and uncontrollable and incontinence is likely.
- The distal clearance margin should be ≥ 2 cm for well differentiated tumours and ≥ 5 cm for poorly differentiated tumours.
- Excision of the mesorectum reduces the incidence of local recurrence of rectal cancer.
- A loop ileostomy may be performed to protect a low anastomosis.
- Subtotal colectomy and ileo-rectal anastomosis is indicated in FAP, Lynch syndrome and younger patients with left-sided obstruction.
- A colonic pouch–anal anastomosis may be performed for very low rectal tumours.
- Chemotherapy. 5-FU and leucovorin are sometimes used in Dukes C. Intraportal 5-FU and heparin for 1 week post-operatively seems to prolong survival in Dukes C. Systemic levamisole is used in the USA.
  - Radiotherapy is indicated in rectal cancer (Dukes B and C). It may be given post-operatively or pre-operatively. It is also useful for inoperable or recurrent cancers.
- Management of locally advanced disease:
  - En-block surgical excision is the mainstay of management.
  - Ureter involvement can be managed with ureteroureterostomy, Boari flap reconstruction, ileal conduit, ureterostomy, spout colostomy diversion or nephrostomy.
  - For rectal cancer radiotherapy may be given pre-operatively to shrink tumours or post-operatively for involved margins.
  - Chemotherapy in the form of systemic 5-FU should be given to fit patients
- Management of liver metastases:
  - Hepatic resection is possible in 25% of cases and the 5 year survival rate is 20% after surgery.
  - Systemic 5-FU and folinic acid may be given for inoperable liver metastases with 30% response rate. Raltitrexed is effective in the palliation of metastatic disease.
- Management of other metastases:
  - Radiotherapy for bony metastases.
  - Radiotherapy and corticosteroids for brain metastases.
- Management of local recurrence:
  - Clinical local recurrence occurs in 10% of cases.

- 70% of patients with local recurrence have distant metastases.
- Treatment modalities include surgical excision, endoluminal excision (using diathermy or laser) and/or radiotherapy.

**Prognosis**

- The 5-year survival rate is 90% for Dukes A, 55% for Dukes B, 30% for Dukes C and 15% for Dukes D.

**Follow Up**

- History and examination (including rigid sigmoidoscopy) is performed every 3 months for the first 3 years and then every 6 months thereafter.
- Serum CEA may be measured regularly.
- Colonoscopic surveillance every 4 years for patients presenting with a single cancer and every 2 years for those presenting with multiple cancers.

# 17. Anal Cancer

## Epidemiology

- The incidence varies from 0.2 (Philippines) per $10^5$ per year to 3.6 (Switzerland) per $10^5$ per year.
- The incidence is increasing world-wide.

## Aetiology

- Risk factors include:
  - Receptive anal intercourse.
  - Human papilloma virus (HPV) type 16, 18, 31 and 33 DNA.
  - Herpes simplex virus type II.
  - *Chlamydia* and HIV infection.

## Pathology

- 80% of lesions are epidermoid and the remainder consists of melanoma and adenocarcinoma.
- Local spread tends to occur in cephalad direction.
- Nodal spread to perirectal, inguinal and lateral pelvic nodes may occur.

## Clinical Features

- Pain and bleeding in 50% of cases.
- Anal mass/ulcer, faecal incontinence and/or ano-vaginal fistula.
- Inguinal lymphadenopathy in 30% of cases (metastases are confirmed in only 50% of such cases).
- Hepatomegaly (uncommon).

## Investigations

- Proctoscopy and biopsy.
- Examination under anaesthetic (EUA) and biopsy.
- Endoanal USS.
- CT or MRI.

**Treatment**

- Combined radiotherapy (50 Gy) and chemotherapy (5-FU and mitomycin C) is the mainstay of management (Nigro's regimen)
- Surgical treatment is indicated for failure of primary non-surgical
  therapy (residual tumour, radionecrosis, fistulae and local recurrence),
  for small lesions at the anal margin and for inguinal recurrence after
  radiotherapy.
- Surgical procedures include abdominoperineal resection, defunctioning
  colostomy, excision of perianal lesions and inguinal node dissection.
- Adenocarcinoma is usually treated with abdominoperineal resection and
  melanoma is treated with more conservative surgery owing to poor prognosis.

**Prognosis**

The overall 5-year survival rate for epidermoid carcinoma is 58% and local
control rate with radiotherapy and chemotherapy is 90%.

# 18. Gall Bladder Cancer

## Epidemiology

- Gall-bladder cancer is found incidentally in 2% of all gall-bladders excised for gallstones.
- The peak incidence occurs during 60–80 years.
- The male:female ratio is 2:5.

## Aetiology

- It is associated with gallstones in 75% of cases.
- Carcinogens including nitrosamines and methylcholanthrene.
- A higher incidence is reported among rubber workers and typhoid carriers.

## Pathology

- The histological subtypes include adenocarcinoma (85%), squamous carcinoma (3%) and undifferentiated (7%).
- The tumour tends to invade locally.
- Spread may occur through the intraductal lymphatic or vascular routes.
- The lesion appears macroscopically as a nodule, polypoid mass or focal/diffuse thickening.

## Clinical Features

- Incidental finding in a cholecystectomy specimen.
- Pain (80%), nausea and vomiting (50%), weight loss (40%), jaundice (40%), abdominal distension (30%), pruritus (15%) and melaena (3%).
- Hepatomegaly (40%), mass in the right hypochondrium (40%) and upper abdominal tenderness (40%).

## Investigations

- FBC and LFTs.
- Ultrasound, CT and/or MRI.

- Cholangiography (ERCP/PTC).

## Nevin's Staging

- Stage I (mucosa only), stage II (mucosa and muscularis), stage III (transmural), stage IV (transmural and cystic lymph node) and stage V (liver invasion/distant metastases).

## Treatment

- Simple open cholecystectomy for stages I and II.
- Radical cholecystectomy including adjacent liver resection and regional lymph node dissection for stage III and IV. Pancreaticoduodenectomy is performed in selected cases. Radical surgery may be performed for stage V in fit patients.
- Palliative procedures include stenting (endoscopic or percutaneous) and surgical bypass (Roux-en-Y hepatico-jejunostomy).
- Intra-operative radiotherapy for stages III, IV and V.

## Prognosis

- The 5-year survival rate is 60% for stage I, 40% for stage II, 10% for stage III, 7% for stage IV and 1% for stage V.

# 19. Cholangiocarcinoma

## Epidemiology

- Accounts for 1.5% of all cancers.
- Commoner in the 6th and 7th decades and among males.

## Aetiology

- Risk factors include:
  - Gallstones (found in 30% of cases).
  - Choledochal cysts.
  - Caroli's disease.
  - Sclerosing cholangitis.
  - Ulcerative colitis.
  - *Clonorchis sinesis* infestation (liver fluke).
  - *Opsithorchis viverrini* infestation.
  - Thorium dioxide and drugs (OCP and methyldopa).

## Pathology

- Common bile duct (CBD) is the commonest location (40%) followed by common hepatic duct (32%), hepatic duct bifurcation (20%) and cystic duct (5%).
- Adenocarcinoma is the commonest type (97%).
- The tumour may be peripheral (type I), hilar (type II), middle third extrahepatic (type III) or distal extrahepatic (type IV).

## Clinical Factors

- Jaundice is the commonest presentation (95%).
- Abdominal pain.
- Hepatomegaly.
- Pruritus.
- Abdominal tenderness.
- Ascites.
- Abnormal LFTs.

**Investigations**

- LFTs.
- Ultrasound, CT and/or MRI scan.
- Cholangiography (ERCP and/or PTC).
- Angiography or Doppler study to assess resectability.


**Treatment and Prognosis**

- Resectable tumours of the distal third of the CBD are treated with radical pancreaticoduodenectomy (Whipple's procedure). The 5-year survival rate is 50%.
- The resectable tumours of the middle third are treated with excision (1 cm clear margin) and biliary-intestinal anastomosis (hepatico-jejun-ostomy). The 5-year survival rate is 50%.
- For proximal hilar tumours 'attempt at cure' surgery has been proposed. The surgery involves local excision alone for type I, local excision and partial hepatectomy for types II and III or orthoptic liver transplantation (OLT) for type IV. The 3-year survival rate is 30%. Resectability rate is 20% (vs 65% for tumours of the middle and distal thirds of the CBD).
- Partial hepatectomy or OLT for peripheral cholangiocarcinoma. The 3-year survival rate is 50%.
- Palliative procedures for unresectable tumours or unfit patients. Proce-dures include stent placement (endoscopic or percutaneous transhepatic) and surgical biliary intestinal anastomosis. Self-expandable stainless steel endoprostheses are to be preferred for palliation. The median survival rate is 8 months.
- Adjuvant therapy. Chemotherapy and radiotherapy have no established role in management as yet.

# 20. Hepatocellular Carcinoma (HCC)

**Epidemiology**

- Commonest primary cancer of the liver.
- Males are more commonly affected (3:2).
- Peak incidence 40–60 years.

**Aetiology**

- Risk factors include:
  - Aflatoxin.
  - Hepatic cirrhosis.
  - Vital hepatitis (B and C).
  - Haemochromatosis.
  - $\alpha_1$-antitrypsin deficiency.
  - Tobacco smoking.
  - Oestrogenic steroids.
  - Autoimmune chronic hepatitis.
  - Primary biliary cirrhosis.
  - Wilson's disease.

**Pathology**

- Diffuse.
- Single.
- Encapsulated.
- Fibrolamellar.

**Clinical Features**

- Pain:
  - Epigastric.
  - Right hypochondrium.
  - Back.
- Anorexia.
- Dyspnoea (lung metastases/pleural effusion).
- Ascites.

- Hepatomegaly.
- Bleeding.
- Oesophageal varices.
- Obstructive jaundice.
- Bony metastases
- Arterial murmur over the tumour.
- Paraneoplastic symptoms include:
  - Fever.
  - Hypoglycaemia.
  - Hypercalcaemia.
  - Polycythaemia.

**Investigations**

- FBC, serum biochemistry and clotting screen.
- Serum α-fetoprotein (AFP) is a useful marker.
- Hepatitis screen (B and C).
- Abdominal (sunburst calcification) and chest X-ray.
- CT scan and ultrasound scan, angiography, Doppler flow studies and/or portal venography.
- FNAC or core biopsy under radiological guidance. Biopsy should be avoided in patients coming to resection or transplantation to avoid tumour spread along needle track.

**Treatment**

- Peripheral wedge resection of small superficial carcinomas.
- Hepatic segmental resection is the mainstay of curative treatment. Patients with multicentric tumours, severe liver impairment, ascites and distant metastases are excluded.
- Orthoptic liver transplantation should be offered to carefully selected patients without dissemination who are not suitable for segmental resection.
- Chemotherapy effective agents include adriamycin, cisplatin and mitozantrone. These drugs may be combined with lipiodol to allow secretive retention within the tumour. Response rate is 45%.
- Arterial embolisation – particularly effective in the management of ruptured HCC:
  - Performed percutaneously using gelfoam, Ivalon, steel coils or starch microspheres.
  - Post-embolisation syndrome consists of pyrexia, pain, nausea and

worsening LFTs.
- Contraindicated in the presence of portal vein thrombosis.
- Percutaneous ethanol injection causes complete necrosis in more than 90% of small tumours (< 3 cm).
- Radiotherapy may be given in the form of external beam radiation, percutaneous injection of radioactive material or transcatheter injection of $[^{131}I]$-lipiodol.
- Tamoxifen is a recognised treatment modality.


**Prognosis**

- The 3-year survival rate for resection is 40%.
- The 3-year survival for transplantation is 25%.
- The 1-year survival for untreated patients is 20%.

# 21. Carcinoma of the Pancreas

## Epidemiology

* The incidence varies from 2 to 15 per 100000 per year depending upon geographic location. The incidence is increasing.
* The female to male ratio is 3:1.
* The peak incidence is 60–80 years.

## Aetiology

Pancreatic cancer is associated with:
* Cigarette smoking (2.5-fold increase in risk).
* High intake of animal fats and coffee.
* Pancreatitis (hereditary or chronic).
* Ataxia telangiectasia.

## Pathology

* The tumour type may be:
  * Ductal (82%).
  * Giant cell (6%).
  * Adenosquamous (4%).
  * Mucinous adenocarcinoma (2%).
  * Mucinous cystadenocarcinoma (1%).
  * Acinar cell carcinoma (1%).

## Clinical Features

* Jaundice (pancreatic head tumours).
* Pain.
* Weight loss.
* Pancreatitis.
* Upper GI haemorrhage.
* Thromboembolic disease.
* Cholangitis.
* Psychiatric disturbance.
* Thrombophlebitis.

- Migraine.
- Upper abdominal mass.
- Constipation.
- Bloating.
- Diarrhoea.
- Fatigue.
- Palpable gall bladder.
- Splenomegaly.
- Hepatomegaly.
- Diabetes mellitus.

**Investigations**

- FBC, serum U&Es, LFTs, clotting screen, ultrasonography, ERCP and CT scanning.
- Brush cytology, FNAC or core biopsy under radiological guidance.
- The staging investigations include:
  - Colour flow doppler ultrasonography.
  - Angiography.
  - Laparoscopy.
  - Endoscopic ultrasonography.
  - Laparotomy.

**Treatment**

- Correction of clotting and electrolyte abnormalities.
- Surgical resection:
  - This is indicated for small tumours (< 3 cm in diameter) and favourable histological types in the absence of distant metastases.
  - It is possible in 50% of patients.
  - Whipple's operation for tumours of the head and distal pancreatectomy for tumours of the body and tail. More radical resection does not improve survival.
  - Whipple's operation entails proximal pancreatectomy, gastroduodenal resection, cholecystectomy, pancreatico-jejunostomy, choledocho-jejunostomy and gastrojejunostomy.
  - The operative mortality rate should be < 5%.
- Palliative surgery:
  - Choledochoduodenostomy and retrocolic gastrojejunostomy.
  - Endoscopic stent placement (self-expanding metal-mesh stents are preferred).

- There is no difference in survival between surgical bypass and stenting.
- Radiotherapy:
  - It may be given adjuvantly after resection.
  - Radiotherapy and 5-FU increase survival in non-resectable tumours.
- Chemotherapy:
  - 5-FU seems to be an effective agent. The objective response rate is 20%.
- Coeliac plexus block for pain palliation.


**Prognosis**

- The median survival after surgical resection is 18 months (higher for mucinous adenocarcinoma).
- The average survival after palliation is 5.4 months.

# 22. Multiple Endocrine Neoplasia (MEN) Syndromes

- MEN I:
  - Autosomal dominant inheritance.
  - Involves pituitary, islet cells of pancreas and parathyroid glands.
  - Thyroid adenomas, carcinoids, adrenal adenomas, thymomas and ovarian tumours are associated with MEN I.
- MEN IIa:
  - Autosomal dominant inheritance.
  - Includes medullary thyroid carcinoma (MTC), phaeochromocytoma and parathyroid adenoma or hyperplasia.
- MEN IIb:
  - Autosomal dominant or sporadic.
  - Includes phaeochromocytoma, MTC, submucosal neuromas, ganglio-neuromas and marfanoid habitus.

# 23. Insulinoma

## Pathology

- Originates in the β-cells of the pancreatic islets.
- 90% of insulinomas are small single adenomas.
- Insulinomas associated with MEN I are multiple in 75% of cases.
- 10% of insulinomas are malignant.

## Clinical Features

- The clinical picture is defined by Whipple's triad:
  - Symptoms and signs of hypoglycaemia occurring during fasting or exercise.
  - At the time of symptoms, the blood glucose level is below 60 mg/dl.
  - The symptoms are reversed by glucose administration.

## Investigations

- Serum insulin:glucose ratio. This usually exceeds 1 in insulinoma patients.
- Localisation using selective venous sampling, angiography, CT and/or MRI.
- Intraoperative USS.
- Provocative tests.

## Treatment

- Small benign lesions can be enucleated.
- Malignant lesions are treated by pancreatic resection (distal pancreatectomy or Whipple's operation). Stropozotocin is an effective chemotherapeutic agent.

## Prognosis

- The median survival for malignant tumours is 5 years after curative resection.

- The median disease-free survival falls to four years after palliative resection.

# 24. Gastrinoma

## Pathology

- A non-β islet cell tumour of the pancreas is the commonest cause.
- 60% of tumours are malignant.
- 65% of cases occur in the pancreas and 35% in the duodenum.
- Gastrinoma is associated with MEN type I.

## Clinical Features

- Causes hypergastrinaemia and hypersecretion of gastric acid (atypical peptic ulceration, Zollinger–Ellison syndrome).

## Investigations

- Serum gastrin and gastric acid output.
- Secretin test.
- Localisation with arteriography, upper gastrointestinal series, CT, selective venous sampling and/or MRI.

## Treatment

- Surgical resection of well-localised tumours. Only 20% of tumours are resectable.
- Medical treatment with: omeprazole, lansoprazole, somatostatin analogues and/or streptozotocin.
- Total gastrectomy is a recognised treatment modality.

# 25.  Malignant Phaeochromocytoma

## Pathology

- Arises from the neural crest-derived chromaffin tissue.
- Accounts for approximately 7% of phaeochromocytomas.
- 90% are found in the adrenal medulla.
- Secretes excess amounts of adrenaline and noradrenaline.

## Clinical Features

- Usually presents with general symptoms such as hypertension, palpitations, headaches, anxiety, nausea and vomiting and local symptoms depending upon location.

## Investigations

- Diagnosis is based on elevated serum and urinary catecholamines (VMA, adrenaline and noradrenaline).
- Neuron-specific enolase is a useful marker.
- Localisation using [$^{131}$I]-MIBG scan (95% accuracy), CT and/or MRI.
- Vena cava sampling is occasionally performed.

## Treatment

- Preoperative preparation includes $\alpha$-blockade (3 weeks of phenoxybenzamine), $\beta_1$-blockade and correction of vascular volume.
- Surgical removal of tumour.
- Embolisation.
- $\alpha$- and $\beta$-blockers for symptom control.
- [$^{131}$I]-MIBG and chemotherapy (cyclophosphamide, vincristine and decarbazine).

## Prognosis

- The 5-year survival rate is 40%.

# 26. Adrenocortical Malignancy

**Epidemiology**

- Incidence is 0.1 per 100 000 per year.
- Women are more commonly affected.
- The peak incidence occurs during the fourth decade.

**Pathology**

- Tumours may be non-functioning (compressing and invading surrounding structures) or functioning causing Cushing's syndrome (50%), virilisation (30%), feminisation (12%) and Conn's syndrome (very rare).
- 40% of patients have metastases at presentation.

**Investigations**

- Biochemical measurement (serum cortisol, ACTH, steroid suppression tests, etc).
- CT, USS, MRI, IVU, angiography and/or selective venous sampling.
- CT-guided biopsy.

**Treatment**

- Adrenalectomy (lateral or anterior approach).
- Chemotherapy (mitotane, streptozotocin, 5-FU, doxorubicin and/or cisplatin).

**Prognosis**

- The 5-year survival is 20%.

# 27. Carcinoid Tumours

## Epidemiology

- Carcinoid tumours arise from APUD (amine precursor uptake decarboxylase) cells and secrete serotonin.
- The incidence is 1.5 per 100 000 per year.

## Pathology

- 75% of the tumours occur in the mid-gut with 45% in the appendix.

## Clinical Features

- Carcinoids present with local symptoms (appendicitis or bowel obstruction) or symptoms of the carcinoid syndrome (found in 9% of cases).
- Right cardiac complications occur in 50% of cases.

## Investigations

- The investigation of choice is 24-hourly urinary 5-hydroxyindole acetic acid (5-HIAA).
- Barium studies, colonoscopy, CT, MRI, USS and/or laparoscopy.

## Management

- Surgery:
    - Appendix: appendicectomy for lesions < 2 cm in size and right hemicolectomy for lesions > 2 cm in size.
    - Stomach and duodenum: local excision for tumours < 1 cm in size.
    - Small bowel: small bowel resection with mesentery.
    - Rectum: local excision if < 2 cm and excision of rectum if the lesion is > 2 cm.
    - Solitary metastasis in liver can be treated by hepatic resection.
- Chemotherapy:
    - The response rate is 33%.
    - 5-FU, stroptozotocin, doxorubicin and cyclophosphamide are usually

       used.
- Embolisation for hepatic metastases.
- Interferons.
- Other drugs include histamine antagonists, 5-HT antagonists and somatostatin analogues.
- Chemotherapy:
  - The response rate is 50%.
  - The role is not clearly defined.
  - It may be given as an adjuvant to surgery and/or radiotherapy.
- Other treatments include:
  - Brachytherapy.
  - Photodynamic therapy.
  - Endoscopic mucosectomy.
  - Surgical bypass (Kirchner operation).
  - Electrocoagulation.
  - Ethanol injection.

**Prognosis**

- The 5-year survival rate is 5%.

# 28. Thyroid Cancer

**Epidemiology**

- The incidence is 3.1 per 100 000 per year.
- The female to male ratio is 2.5:1.

**Aetiology**

- Radiation (accounts for 10% of cases).
- Genetic factors (medullary thyroid carcinoma – MTC).
- Pre-existing benign conditions (e.g. Hashimoto's thyroiditis, multi-nodular and endemic goitres).

**Pathology**

- Papillary tumours:
  - These tumours account for 70% of cases.
  - The tumours are usually low grade.
  - The incidence of multifocal and bilateral disease is 80%.
  - The regional lymph nodes are involved in 50% of cases.
- Follicular tumours:
  - These tumours account for 16% of cases.
  - Lymph node metastases occur in 5% of cases.
  - Vascular invasion is a poor prognostic indicator.
  - Hurtle cell carcinoma is a cytological variant of follicular carcinoma.
- Medullary tumours:
  - These tumours account for 6% of cases.
  - These tumours arise in parafollicular C-cells.
  - There is an association with MEN syndrome (type IIA).
  - Calcitonin is a useful serum marker.
  - The tumours may secrete ACTH and prostaglandins.
- Anaplastic carcinoma:
  - It accounts for 7% of cases.
  - It occurs predominantly in the elderly and carries a poor prognosis.
- Lymphoma:
  - Accounts for 1% of thyroid tumours.
  - It is usually the non-Hodgkin's type.
  - Poor prognostic indicators include spread beyond cervical nodes, necrosis and vascular invasion.

**Clinical Presentation**

- Incidental pathological findings in a thyroidectomy specimen excised for benign disease.
- Discrete thyroid nodule.
- Recently enlarging multinodular goitre.
- Cervical lymphadenopathy.
- Neck mass with pressure symptoms.
- Voice change.
- Distant metastases.

**Investigations**

- Fine needle aspiration cytology. This is the most useful investigation.
- Thyroid function tests.
- Ultrasonography.
- Core biopsy.
- CXR.
- CT.
- MRI.
- Radioactive iodine scan.
- Serum calcitonin.

**Management**

- Total thyroidectomy and removal of involved lymph nodes. The recurrent laryngeal nerve should be identified and preserved. Attempts should be made to preserve the parathyroids.
- Thyroxine in order to suppress thyroid stimulating hormone (TSH).
- Radioactive iodine ($[^{131}I]$) for follicular carcinoma, advanced papillary carcinoma (stages II to IV) and metastatic disease.
- External beam radiation for inadequately excised papillary, follicular, medullary and Hurtle cell carcinomas.
- External radiation and chemotherapy are used to control anaplastic carcinoma.
- Lymphoma is treated by radiotherapy. Chemotherapy is indicated if there is retrosternal or distant spread.

**Follow Up**

- Physical examination
- Thyroid function tests.
- Serum thyroglobulin.
- Radioactive iodine [$^{131}$I] scan.
- Serum calcitonin (medullary carcinoma).

**Prognosis**

- Papillary carcinoma:
  - Low grade tumours: the 20-year survival is 93%.
  - Locally invasive tumour: the 15-year survival is 15%.
- Follicular carcinoma:
  - Medullary carcinoma: the 5-year survival rate is 55%.
  - Anaplastic carcinoma: the 3-year survival rate is 3%.

**Screening for MTH**

- First degree relatives of patients with MTC should be screened for MTC and other endocrine neoplasms such as parathyroid adenoma and phaeo-chromocytoma.
- Screening for MTC includes physical examination, serum calcitonin, PTH, VMA, cytogenetics and biopsy.
- Medullary thyroid hyperplasia is a premalignant condition and is a recognised indication for prophylactic total thyroidectomy.

# 29. Parathyroid Carcinoma

**Epidemiology**

- Accounts for 1% of al cases of primary hyperthyroidism.
- Equal sex distribution.

**Pathology**

- Histological diagnosis is often difficult.
- Chief cells predominate.
- Flow cytometric analysis of DNA aids the diagnosis.

**Presentation**

- Symptoms of hypercalcaemia including renal stones (56%) and bone involvement (90%).
- Acute pancreatitis (12% of cases).
- Neck mass (45% of cases).

**Investigations**

- Serum calcium and parathyroid hormone (higher than in benign disease).
- FNAC.
- Localisation with CT, MRI or thallium–technetium scanning.

**Treatment**

- Treatment of hypercalcaemia (rehydration and biphosphonates).
- *En bloc* removal of the tumour with the thyroid lobe, lymph nodes and ipsilateral isthmus.
- The nerve may be sacrificed if involved.
- Most patients require oral calcium and vitamin D.

## Prognosis

- Frequent measurement of serum calcium and PTH is required during follow up.
- The 5-year survival is 50%.
- The 5-year local recurrence rate is 45%.

# 30. Soft Tissue Sarcoma (STS)

## Epidemiology

- STSs account for 1% of adult cancers and for 15% of paediatric cancers.
- The sex distribution is approximately equal.
- 43% of cases arise in the lower extremity, 16% in the upper extremity, 13% in the visceral organs, 12% in the retroperitoneum, 10% in the trunk, 5% in the head and neck and 3% in the chest.

## Aetiology

- The aetiology is unknown in most cases.
- The risk factors include genetic disorders (Li–Fraumeni syndrome, hereditary retinoblastoma, neurofibromatosis and Gardner's syndrome), radiation, lymphoedema, thorium oxide (angiosarcoma) and vinyl chloride.

## Pathology

- The likelihood of metastasising is > 50% for high-grade sarcomas compared with < 15% for low-grade sarcomas.
- Immunohistochemical analysis (using a panel of antibodies) is used to specify sarcoma type.
- Lymph node metastases occur in < 35% of cases.

## Clinical Features

- Extremity sarcomas present as a painless mass. The presence of pain indicates a poor prognosis.
- Retroperitoneal sarcoma patients present with abdominal mass, abdominal pain, neurological symptoms or bowel obstruction.
- Other symptoms include abnormal uterine bleeding (uterine sarcoma), haematuria (bladder sarcoma) and nasal bleeding/obstruction (nasal and paranasal sarcomas).

**Treatment**

- Extremity and trunk. Limb-sparing surgery is an important principle of treatment.
  - Low-grade tumours of the trunk and extremity are treated by a wide local resection. External radiotherapy is indicated for large (> 5 cm) or incompletely excised tumours.
  - High-grade tumours are treated by a wide local resection followed by adjuvant radiotherapy (brachytherapy/external radiotherapy). Chemotherapy may be considered for large high grade sarcomas (> 10 cm). Lung metastases should be excluded prior to treatment.
- Retroperitoneal and visceral sarcomas are treated by surgical resection. Incompletely excised tumours and large (> 10 cm) high grade tumours should be considered for radiotherapy and chemotherapy.
- Gastrointestinal sarcomas may cause bleeding, perforation, ulceration and/or obstruction. These complications require appropriate surgical treatment.
- A minimal 2 cm margin of normal tissue is required for adequate excision.

**Investigations**

- LFTs, serum U&Es and FBC.
- FNAC (unhelpful), core biopsy, incisional and excisional biopsy.
- MRI scan (superior to CT).
- CXR.
- Thoracic CT if CXR suggests the presence of metastases.
- US or CT of liver.

**Notes**

- Pulmonary metastases can be excised surgically provided there is a good local control of the primary tumour and there is no evidence of extrapulmonary metastases. The 5-year survival rate is 26% following resection.
- Metastatic sarcoma can be treated by chemotherapy (e.g. doxorubicin and ifisoformide) with response rates approaching 35%.
- Local recurrence is treated by surgical excision and radiotherapy.

**Follow Up**

- Patients with high-grade tumours of the extremity and trunk should be examined and have a CXR every 3 months for the first 3 years, twice a year for 2 years and then annually thereafter. A thoracic CT may be performed.
- Patients with visceral and retroperitoneal sarcomas should also have abdominal CT during follow up.


**Prognosis**

- Depends upon size, grade, site, adequacy of excision and histopathological type.
- The 5-year survival rate is 25% for retroperitoneal sarcoma and 80% for extremity sarcoma.

# 31. Kaposi's Sarcoma

**Epidemiology**

- Kaposi's sarcoma (KS) is relatively common among elderly men (> 50 years) of Mediterranean origin, Ashkenasi Jews and persons infected with herpes simplex virus (HSV).
- It is the commonest tumour associated with AIDS.

**Aetiology**

- The risk factors include:
  - HSV infection.
  - Cytomegalovirus infection.
  - Immunosuppression.

**Pathology**

- The tumour is derived from vascular or lymphatic endothelium.

**Clinical Features**

- Pigmented, non-blanching skin lesions. The lesions are initially red/blue and flat, later they become purple, raised and coalescent. There may be associated bruising and/or lymphoedema.
- Mucocutaneous lesions. Intra-oral lesions account for 15% of clinical presentations.
- Gastrointestinal KS may cause GI bleeding, perforation, intussusception and/or obstruction.
- Pulmonary KS may cause dyspnoea, haemoptysis and/or cough.

**Investigations**

- Surgical biopsy.
- HIV testing.
- CD4 count.

**Treatment**

- Radiotherapy for lesions on the face, trunk, limbs and penis. The response rate is 60%.
- Intralesional vinblastine is a recognised treatment modality.
- Camouflaging cream.
- Systemic bleomycin, vincristine and steroids for aggressive skin lesions and symptomatic visceral and pulmonary lesions.
- Zidovudine for the HIV-infected individuals.
- Surgery for the complications of visceral lesions.

**Prognosis**

- Depends on CD4 count, performance status and the presence of multiple lesions.
- The median survival is 1.5 years from the time of diagnosis.

# 32. Osteosarcoma

**Epidemiology**

- It accounts for 3.5% of childhood malignancies.
- It is the commonest primary malignancy of bone.
- The peak incidence occurs in the second decade.
- The male to female ratio is 1.5:1.

**Aetiology**

- Ionising radiation.
- Genetic causes include Li–Fraumeni syndrome, p53 gene and Rb gene.
- Paget's disease of bone.

**Pathology**

- The tumour usually arises in the epiphysis around the knee (lower femur and upper tibia).

**Clinical Features**

- Pain and swelling around the knee. The swelling is usually tender and warm. There may be limitation of limb movement.
- The plain radiograph usually shows a destructive lesion in the metaphyseal region with new bone formation. There may be elevation of the periosteum (Codman's triangle).

**Investigations**

- CT or MRI of the tumour.
- CXR, serum alkaline phosphatase (reflects disease activity), CT of thorax and radio isotope bone scan.

**Management**

- Based on chemotherapy–surgery–chemotherapy:
  - Pre-operative chemotherapy (cisplatin, doxorubicin, ifosfamide and high dose methotrexate for 6–9 weeks).
  - Conservative limb sparing surgery and endoprosthesis.
  - Post-operative chemotherapy for 9–18 weeks using the same agents as in the pre-operative period.
  - Pulmonary metastases are initially treated by chemotherapy to be followed by surgical excision if there is no evidence of further metastases 3 months after chemotherapy.

**Prognosis**

- The overall cure rate is 60%.

# 33.  Cutaneous Melanomas

## Epidemiology

- The incidence varies from 0.7 (black Americans) to 40 (white Australians) per $10^5$ per annum.
- The incidence is rising (50% rise in the last decade)
- The peak incidence occurs during the fifth decade.

## Aetiology

- The risk factors include:
  - Family history of melanoma.
  - History of multiple atypical naevi.
  - The presence of atypical or numerous naevi.
  - Inability to tan.
  - Excessive exposure to ultraviolet radiation.
  - Immunosuppression.
  - Genetic factors such as p53.

## Classification

- Superficial spreading melanoma accounts for 70% of cases.
- Nodular melanoma accounts for 15% of cases.
- Lentigo maligna is uncommon and carries an excellent prognosis.
- Acral lentiginous melanoma makes up 10% of all melanomas.
- Amelanotic melanoma.

## Current Staging System

- IA    Primary melanoma ≤ 0.75 mm thick.
- IB    Primary melanoma 0.7–1.5 mm thick.
- IIA   Primary melanoma 1.5–4 mm thick.
- IIB   Primary melanoma ≥ 4 mm in thickness.
- III   The presence of regional nodal involvement or in-transit lesions.
- IV    The presence of systemic metastases.

**Investigations**

- Incisional or excisional biopsy. The latter is to be preferred if possible.
- FNAC of masses suggestive of metastases, e.g. regional lymph nodes.
- Staging investigations include CXR, liver USS, CT and bone scan.

**Treatment**

- Primary melanoma is treated by adequate local excision. The defect is closed primarily or using skin grafts and local flaps. The clear margins should be 1 cm for thicknesses < 2 mm and 2 cm for thicknesses 2–4 mm.
- Lymph nodes:
  - Elective lymph node dissection is performed if the primary melanoma > 1.5 mm thick and/or there is lymph node involvement.
  - Alternatively, a regional lymph node dissection is performed if the sentinel node is positive for metastatic disease. The sentinel node can be accurately identified using scintigraphy and provides an accurate assessment of the regional lymph nodes.
  - The pattern of lymphatic drainage may be determined by using lymphatic scintigraphy.
- High-dose interferon-$\alpha$ seems to improve survival in patients with high-risk melanoma.
- Locally advanced/recurrent melanoma is treated by hyperthermic isolated limb perfusion (e.g. melphalan) with a remission rate of 40%.
- Distant metastases:
  - Systemic chemotherapy using decarbazine (20–25% response rate).
  - Solitary or limited numbers of metastases in the brain, intestine or lungs can be resected with prolongation of survival.
  - Immunotherapy, e.g. interferon-$\alpha$ and vaccination, are still under investigation.
  - Radiotherapy for palliation of inoperable brain, lymph nodes and bone metastases.

**Follow Up**

- Stage IA patients should be reviewed 6 monthly for 2 years, then yearly.
- Stage IB and II patients should be reviewed 4 monthly for 3 years, then yearly.
- Stage IIB and III patients should be reviewed 4 monthly for 5 years then yearly.
- Patients are educated in self-examination.

## Prognosis

- Depends upon tumour stage, ulceration, age, sex, primary lesion site and growth pattern.
- The 5-year survival rate is 95% for stage IA, 85% for stage IB, 55% for stage IIA, 40% for stage IIB, 30% for stage III and < 1% for stage IV.

# 34. Non-melanocytic Skin Cancer

## Epidemiology

- This is the commonest cancer among Caucasians in the UK and USA.
- The incidence is increasing.
- The incidence is slightly higher in men (especially after the age of 70 years).

## Aetiology

- Actinic radiation.
- Chronic skin ulcers and sinuses,
- Immunosuppression.
- Genetic predisposition, e.g. xeroderma pigmentosum, multiple familial self-healing squamous carcinoma and Gorlin Goltz syndrome (basal cell carcinoma).
- Bowen's disease predisposes to squamous cell carcinoma.

## Pathology

- Basal cell carcinoma (BCC) usually invades locally. Regional lymph node involvement is extremely rare.
- Squamous cell carcinoma (SCC) systemic spread occurs in 2% of cases.

## Clinical Features

- A skin ulcer. The ulcer margins may be rolled (SCC) or pearly and everted (BCC). Surface telangiectasia may be present (BCC).
- A skin nodule or cystic lesion.
- The skin lesion is occasionally pigmented.
- Regional lymphadenopathy (SCC).

## Investigations

- Excisional biopsy.
- Incisional biopsy.

- Shaving biopsy.
- FNAC of enlarged lymph nodes.

## Treatment

- Adequate surgical excision with a minimal margin of 4 mm for BCC and 1 cm for SCC. The surgical defect can be closed primarily or using a skin graft, a local flap or myocutaneous flap (conventional or free transfer).
- Radiotherapy is an effective treatment modality.
- Regional lymph node dissection or radiotherapy for involved nodes.
- Other treatment modalities include cryosurgery, laser, curettage or electro-desiccation.

## Prognosis

- The 5-year survival is 98% for SCC and 100% for BCC.
- Death from BCC is extremely rare.
- The 5-year incidence of further BCC lesions is 40%.

# 35.  Ovarian Cancer

## Epidemiology

- Ovarian cancer accounts for 25% of all gynaecological malignancies.
- The incidence is 17 per $10^5$ per annum.
- Peak incidence occurs during 40–60 years of life.

## Aetiology

- The risk factors include:
  - Late menopause.
  - Family history of ovarian, endometrial, breast or bowel cancer.
  - Nulliparity.
  - Late first pregnancy.
  - Peritoneal talc use.
  - BRCA-1 gene.

## Pathology

- Epithelial carcinoma accounts for 90% of cases.
- Exfoliation through the peritoneal cavity and lymphatic spread are the commonest modes of dissemination.

## Clinical Features

- Irregular periods.
- Abnormal vaginal bleeding.
- Abdominal pain.
- Urinary or bowel symptoms.
- Ascites.
- Abdominal distension.
- Dyspareunia and anorexia.
- Pelvic mass.

## Investigations

- Abdomino-pelvic US, CT or MRI scan.
- Serum CA125, α-feta protein (AFP) and human chorionic gonado-trophin (HCG).
- CXR, IVU and barium enema.
- Laparoscopy.
- Laparotomy/biopsies.

## Treatment

- Early stage disease confined to the ovary can be treated by total abdominal hysterectomy and bilateral salpingo-oophrectomy (BSO), infracolic omentectomy and surgical staging. Systemic chemotherapy is required for grade 3 tumours.
- Advanced stage disease is treated by debulking surgery aiming to reduce the disease to < 1.5 cm tumour followed by chemotherapy (cisplatinum and cyclophosphamide for 6 cycles).
- Recurrent disease is treated by chemotherapy (e.g. Taxol) and/or radio-therapy.
- Germ cell tumours in the young are treated by chemotherapy following surgical staging.

## Prognosis

- The 5-year survival rate is 88% for stage I lesions (lesions confined to the ovary), 70% for stage II (lesions extending to the pelvis only) and 20% for advanced disease.

# 36. Endometrial Carcinoma

## Epidemiology

- Endometrial carcinoma is the commonest gynaecological malignancy.
- The median age is 60 years.
- 20% of cases occur before the menopause.
- The incidence is low in Nigeria (0.6 per $10^5$ women) and high in the UK (14 per $10^5$ women).

## Aetiology

- Risk factors include:
  - Obesity.
  - Late menopause.
  - Diabetes mellitus.
  - Nulliparity.
  - Unopposed oestrogen exposure.
  - Tamoxifen therapy.

## Pathology

- Adenocarcinoma is the commonest type (90%).
- Other histopathological types include adenocanthoma, adenosquamous and leiomyosarcoma.
- Direct extension is the commonest mode of spread.

## Clinical Features

- Abnormal vaginal bleeding (90% of cases).
- Abnormal cervical smear cytology.
- Symptoms and signs of metastases.

## Investigations

- Cervical smear cytology and endocervical curettage.
- Endometrial biopsy.

- Dilatation and curettage.
- Hysteroscopy.
- Staging investigations include FBC, LFTs, U&Es, CXR, IVP, abdomino-pelvic CT or MRI and/or bone scan (if indicated).

## Staging (FIGO)

- Stage I:
  - Ia: Tumour limited to the endometrium.
  - Ib: Invasion < 50% of myometrium.
  - Ic: Invasion > 50% of myometrium.
- Stage II:
  - IIa: Endocervical glandular involvement only.
  - IIb: Cervical stromal invasion.
- Stage III:
  - IIIa: Tumour invades serosa/positive peritoneal washings.
  - IIIb: Vaginal metastases.
  - IIIc: Metastases to pelvic/aortic lymph nodes.
- Stage IV:
  - IVa: Invasion of bowel/bladder mucosa.
  - IVb: Distant metastases.

## Treatment

- Stage I and II disease is treated by total abdominal hysterectomy and bilateral salpingo-oophorectomy (BSO). Pelvic and para-aortic lymph nodes are sampled. Radiotherapy is indicated for poorly differentiated carcinoma (garde III).
- Stage Ic, IIA and IIb lesions. Large stage I lesions may be treated by pre-operative radiotherapy followed by hysterectomy and BSO 6 weeks later.
- Advanced and recurrent lesions are treated by a combination of surgery, radiotherapy, chemotherapy (doxorubicin) and hormonal manipulation.
- Hormonal manipulation includes megestrol acetate (80 mg bd), medroxy-progesterone acetate (50 mg tds) and anti-oestrogens.

## Prognosis

- The 5-year survival rate is 73% for stage I, 56% for stage II, 30% for stage III and 10% for stage IV.

# 37. Cervical Cancer

## Epidemiology

- This disease ranks eighth among cancers in women.
- 13 500 new cases are diagnosed in the USA every year.
- The average age is 45 years.
- The incidence is declining.

## Aetiology

- The risk factors include cervical intraepithelial neoplasia (CIN), young age at first intercourse, high parity, low socio-economic status, human papilloma virus (HPV) infection (types 16, 18, 31, 33 and 35), smoking, venereal infections and multiple sexual partners.

## Pathology

- Squamous cell carcinoma (SCC) accounts for 80% of cases.
- Adenocarcinoma and adenosquamous lesions account for 20% of cases.

## Clinical Features

- Vaginal discharge.
- Abnormal vaginal bleeding (post-coital, post-menopausal or irregular) is present in 85% of cases.
- Abnormal routine cervical smear.
- The cervical tumour may be ulcerative, necrotic, exophytic or granular in appearance.
- Pelvic mass.
- Ureteric obstruction in advanced disease.
- Signs and symptoms of metastases, e.g. ascites and inguinal lymphadenopathy.

## Investigations

- Colposcopy plus biopsy, endocervical curettage or conniption.

- Cystoscopy and IVP.
- Sigmoidoscopy/barium enema.
- CXR (lung metastases are present in 5% of cases).
- Abdomino-pelvic CT or MRI scan.
- Bone scan.
- Combined vaginal and rectal examination under anaesthesia.
- FBC, serum U&Es and LFTs.

## Staging (FIGO)

- Stage O:   Carcinoma *in situ.*
- Stage I:   Carcinoma is confined to the cervix.
- Stage II:  Carcinoma extends beyond the cervix, but has not extended to the pelvic wall or the lower third of the vagina.
- Stage III: Carcinoma has extended to the pelvic wall or the lower third of the vagina.
- Stage IV:  Carcinoma has extended beyond the pelvic wall or has involved the rectal/vesical mucosa clinically.
- Stage IVb: Carcinoma is palliated by radiotherapy and chemotherapy.

## Treatment

- CIN is managed by colposcopy and cryosurgery, $CO_2$ laser, electrocoagulation, loop electrodiathermy or cervical conization. CIN II may be cured by hysterectomy in patients who have completed childbearing.
- Microinvasive disease (Stage Ia) can be treated by a cone biopsy (with clear margins) or extrafascial abdominal hysterectomy.
- Stage Ib and IIa tumours are treated by radical hysterectomy with excision of parametrical tissue, vaginal cuff, lymphadenectomy and sampling of the para-aortic nodes or radiotherapy (external beam followed by intracavity radiation).
- Stage IIb, IIa and IIB lesions are treated by radiotherapy (external beam followed by intracavity radiotherapy).
- Stage IVa carcinoma is treated by pelvic radiotherapy. Salvage pelvic extenteration is reserved for partially responding tumours.
- Recurrent disease is treated by chemotherapy (mitomycin C, methotrexate, cyclophosphamide, bleomycin and cis-platinum), pelvic extenteration and/or radiotherapy.

**Prognosis**

- The 5-year survival rate is 75% for stage I, 55% for stage II, 30% for stage III and 7% for stage IV lesions.


**Screening**

- All women, once they have become sexually active, should undergo an annual physical examination and Papanicolaou smear of the cervix.
- The false-negative rate for cervical cytology is 15% and the false positive rate is < 1%.

# 38. Vaginal Cancer

**Epidemiology**

- Primary vaginal cancer accounts for 1.5% of all gynaecological malignancies.
- The highest incidence occurs during 50–70 years of age.
- Most lesions occur in the upper third of the vagina.

**Aetiology**

- Maternal ingestion of diethylstilboestrol during pregnancy increases the incidence of vaginal clear-cell carcinoma in daughters.
- Vaginal intra-epithelial neoplasia has a premalignant potential.
- Other risk factors include:
  - Vaginal pessaries.
  - Venereal disease.
  - HPV infection.
  - Procidentia.
  - Ulceration.
  - Cervical cancer.

**Pathology**

- Squamous cell carcinoma (SCC) accounts for 93% of cases and adeno-carcinoma for 5% of cases.
- Embryonal rhabdomyosarcomas are seen in children.

**Clinical Features**

- Vaginal bleeding/discharge.
- Ulcerative/exophytic vaginal lesions.
- Urinary and gastrointestinal symptoms are occasionally seen.
- Regional lymphadenopathy (inguinal, femoral and obturator).
- Abnormal cervical smear.

## Investigations

- Punch biopsy.
- Colposcopy and endometrial curettage.
- CXR.
- Cystoscopy and IVP.
- Abdomino-pelvic CT or MRI scanning.
- Sigmoidoscopy and/or barium enema.
- FNAC of enlarged lymph nodes.

## Staging (FIGO)

- Stage I:   Tumour confined to the vaginal wall.
- Stage II:  Tumour has involved subvaginal tissue but has not extended to the pelvic wall.
- Stage III: Tumour has extended to the pelvic wall.
- Stage IV:  Tumour has extended beyond the pelvic wall or has involved rectal or vesicle mucosa.

## Treatment

- Radiotherapy (external beam radiation or interstitial) is the mainstay of management. The groins are included in the radiotherapy field for tumours arising in the lower third of the vagina.
- Surgery in the form of a wide local excision or total vaginectomy is indicated for early vaginal cancer. Radical surgery may entail hysterectomy and pelvic lymphadenopathy.
- Psychological counselling is essential prior to vaginectomy.
- A neovagina may be reconstructed using a split thickness skin graft.
- Surgery is indicated for recurrent tumours following radiotherapy.

## Prognosis

- The 5-year survival rate is 87% for stage I, 60% for stage II, 33% for stage III and 7% for stage IV tumours. 10% of patients develop significant bowel and bladder side effects following radiotherapy.

# 39. Vulval Cancer

## Epidemiology

- Vulval cancer accounts for 4% of all gynaecological cancers.
- Highest incidence occurs during the 7th decade of life.

## Aetiology

- The risk factors include immunosuppression, vulval dystrophy and human papilloma virus infection.

## Pathology

- Squamous cell carcinoma accounts for 85% of cases.
- Melanoma accounts for 5% of cases.

## Clinical Features

- Vulval pruritus/pain.
- Vulval ulcer/mass.
- Inguinal lymphadenopathy.

## Investigations

- Surgical biopsy.
- FNAC of regional lymph nodes (if enlarged).
- Abdomino-pelvic CT or MRI for staging.

## Treatment

- Carcinoma *in situ* and microinvasive disease are managed by local vulval excision with a clear margin of 1 cm.
- Lateral cancers < 2 cm in diameter are managed by vulvectomy (with a 2 cm clear margin) and ipsilateral lymph node dissection. A contralateral lymph node dissection is recommended if the ipsilateral nodes are

involved.
- Bilateral inguinal lymph node dissection is indicated for vulval cancer involving the clitoris.
- Pelvic lymphadenectomy is recommended for lesions >4cm in diameter.
- The terminal urethra can be excised in order to achieve adequate local excision.
- Butterfly or triple incision is used for vulvectomy and inguinal node dissection. Skin flaps are created to relieve tension. Deep-vein thrombosis (DVT) and antimicrobial prophylaxis is essential.
- Compression stockings and lymphoedema play an important role after inguinal node dissection (the incidence of lymphoedema is 60%).
- Radiotherapy can be given pre-operatively to render large lesions operable, other indications include inadequate margins and recurrent disease.
- Chemotherapy has a minor role (bleomycin and methotrexate).

# 40. Renal Adenocarcinoma

## Epidemiology

- It accounts for 3% of all adult cancers.
- The male to female ratio is 2:1.
- The peak incidence occurs during 40–60 years of age.

## Aetiology

- The risk factors include Hippel–Lindau syndrome, smoking, exposure to cadmium and polycystic kidneys of patients on renal dialysis.

## Pathology

- Polygonal or round cells with abundant cytoplasm are characteristic.
- Haematogenous spread is the principal mode of metastasis.

## Clinical Features

- The main symptoms are loin pain (40%), haematuria (40%), abdominal mass (25%) and weight loss (35%).
- Other features include varicocele, hypercalcaemia, polycythaemia, hypertension and night sweating.

## Investigations

- Urine microscopy and culture, FBC, serum, U&Es, serum calcium and CXR.
- IVU.
- Ultrasonography.
- CT or MRI scanning.
- Bone scan.

**Treatment**

- Total nephrectomy with perinephric fat and Gerota's fascia after early control and division of renal vessels through an anterior approach.
- Partial nephrectomy for small cortical tumours and bilateral lesions.
- Palliation of metastatic disease includes analgesia, Provera 100 mg tds, radiotherapy to bone secondaries and radiological embolisation for intractable haematuria.
- Interferons and interleukin-2 remain experimental.

**Prognosis**

- The 5-year survival rate is 70% if the tumour is confined within the capsule, 45% if the tumour has breached Gerota's fascia and 30% if there is regional lymph node involvement.

# 41. Wilms' Tumour

## Epidemiology

- It accounts for 6% of all childhood malignancies.
- The peak incidence occurs between 3 and 4 years.

## Pathology

- It may be multifocal and bilateral (5%).
- Mesodermal, mesonephric and metanephric origins have been proposed for this tumour.

## Clinical Features

- Abdominal mass, anorexia, haematuria and/or hypertension.
- Associated congenital abnormalities include aniridia, hemihypertrophy, cryptorchidism and Beckwith syndrome.

## Investigations

- Abdominal USS or CT.
- CXR.
- Renogram.
- Doppler examination of the renal vein and inferior vena cava.

## Staging

- Stage I:   Tumour is confined to the kidney and completely excised.
- Stage II:  Tumour extends beyond renal capsule but completely excised.
- Stage III: Tumour is inoperable, incompletely excised or ruptured diffusely during removal.
- Stage IV:  Distant metastases are present.
- Stage V:   Tumour is bilateral.

**Treatment**

- Surgical debulking of tumour if possible (nephrectomy).
- Chemotherapy and radiotherapy – vincristine and actinomycin D for stages I and II, vincristine, actinomycin and adriamycin for stages III, IV and V.
- Chemotherapy is given preoperatively in stages IV and V.
- Radiotherapy is indicated in stages III, IV and V disease.

**Prognosis**

- The 5-year survival rate is 95% for stages I and II, 82% for stage III, 60% for stage IV and 67% for stage V.

# 42.  Urothelial Carcinoma

## Epidemiology

- The incidence is 17 per $10^5$ per annum.
- The male to female ratio is 3:1.
- It is commoner in industrialised countries.

## Aetiology

- The risk factors include smoking and occupational hazards (rubber, aniline dye, plastics, tyre destruction and cable production).
- Genetic abnormalities and oncogenes (ras and C-myc) have been implicated.
- Balkan nephropathy.
- Drugs, e.g. phenacetin and cyclophosphamide.

## Pathology

- 95% of lesions affect the bladder.
- Transitional cell carcinomas (TCC) can be subdivided into carcinoma *in situ* (CIS), superficial and deep disease (involving muscle).

## Clinical Features

- Haematuria is the commonest symptom.
- Other symptoms include loin pain, urinary tract infection, weight loss, back pain and jaundice.
- Signs include renal and pelvic masses.

## Investigations

- Urine microscopy and culture.
- Urine cytology.
- IVU and flexible cystoscopy.
- Diagnostic cystoscopy (under general anaesthetic) and biopsy.
- USS, CT or MRI.

- Other investigations include LFTs, bone scan, CXR and laparoscopic sampling of pelvic lymph nodes.
- Elderly patients are offered radical cystectomy. The 5-year survival rate is 40%.
- Patients with metastases are treated palliatively. Palliation including radiotherapy, chemotherapy and/or cystectomy. The 2-year survival rate is 5%.
- Catheterisable or continent neobladder (e.g. hemi-Koch pouch) is usually constructed after radical cystectomy.
- Radical cystectomy entails the removal of the prostate, regional lymph nodes, the uterus and anterior vaginal wall.


**Treatment and Prognosis**

- TCC of renal pelvis and ureter is treated by radical nephroureterectomy if the tumour is poorly differentiated or has invaded muscle. Segmental resection and end-to-end anastomosis is suitable for well-differentiated and superficial tumours. Urethroscopic laser may be used to treat small tumours. The median survival is 1 year for invasive tumours and 7 years for non-invasive tumours.
- Superficial TCC is treated by endoscopic transurethral resection and surveillance.
- Intravesical chemotherapy (mitomycin and epirubicin) and immuno-therapy (BCG – bacillus Calmette–Guérin) are suitable for frequent and numerous recurrences.
- Radical cystectomy is considered for high-grade tumours with lamina propria invasion particularly if there is co-existent CIS.
- Primary CIS of the bladder is treated with intravesical mitomycin and BCG in order to prevent aggressive disease. Recurrence or failure to respond to the above treatment is an indication for cystectomy.
- Invasive TCC of the bladder

# 43. Prostatic Adenocarcinoma

**Epidemiology**

- The incidence is 75 per $10^5$ per annum.
- A male has a 10% lifetime risk of developing the disease and a 3% risk of dying from it.
- The incidence is relatively high among American negroes and is low in Japan.

**Aetiology**

- Genetic and environmental factors have been implicated.

**Pathology**

- Most carcinomas arise in the peripheral zone.
- Haematogenous spread occurs predominantly to bone (sclerotic lesions) and lymphatic spread occurs to pelvic nodes.

**Clinical Features**

- Bladder outflow obstruction (urgency, frequency, nocturia, urinary retention and hesitancy).
- Incidental findings in TURP specimens.
- Mass on digital rectal examination.
- Bony pain due to metastases.
- Haematuria.

**Investigations**

- Serum PSA (normal levels < 4 ng/ml). PSA is elevated in prostatic cancer, BPH, prostatitis and urinary retention. It is useful in indicating recurrence (after prostatectomy) and bony metastases.
- Transrectal ultrasonography and biopsy.
- Bone scan and pelvic CT and/or MRI may be indicated.

**Treatment and Prognosis**

- Total prostatectomy
- This is indicated for tumours confined to the prostate.
- The procedure cures all impalpable lesions confined to the prostate (T1) and 35% of palpable tumours which appear to be confined to the prostate (T2).
- The incidence of incontinence should be < 5% and that of impotence < 20%. The incidence of impotence is higher if a nerve-sparing technique is not adopted.
- Radiotherapy (external beam or interstitial):
  - This is indicated for tumours confined to the prostate (T1 and T2). The 5-year survival rate is approximately 65–70%.
  - It is also used to palliate bony pain due to metastases and prostatic bleeding.
- Hormonal manipulation:
  - This is indicated for metastatic disease. 80% of tumours are sensitive to androgen deprivation.
  - Modalities available include diethylstilboestrol (1 mg daily), bicalutamide, cyproterone acetate, flutamide, luteinising hormone-releasing hormone analogues (e.g. goserelin) and orchidectomy (subcapsular or total). These modalities can be used singly or in combination.
  - The median survival for metastatic disease is 30 months.

# 44. Testicular Cancer

## Epidemiology

- The incidence is rising (8 per $10^5$ per year in Denmark).
- The peak incidence occurs between 20–34 years of age.
- The lifetime risk (in Caucasians) is 0.2%.
- The incidence rate is lower among Asians.

## Aetiology

- Risk factors include:
  - Cryptorchidism.
  - Oestrogen exposure.
  - Testicular torsion.
  - Mumps.
  - Orchitis.
  - Testicular trauma.
  - Infertility.
  - Early puberty.
  - Lack of exercise.
  - Orchidectomy.
  - Low sperm counts.
  - Elevated follicle stimulating hormone (FSH).
- It is likely that the FSH-driven overstimulation of spermatogonia is the underlying mechanism for some of the above factors.

## Pathology

- Testicular germ-cell tumours account for 95% of cases.
- Histological subclasses include spermatocytic seminoma (classical and anaplastic), teratoma (differentiated, intermediate and undifferentiated), embryonal carcinoma, choriocarcinoma (pure and mixed) and yolk sac tumour.
- Carcinoma *in situ* (CIS) is a universal precursor.

**Clinical Features**

- Scrotal mass (painless in 75% of cases).
- Solid mass which cannot be distinguished from the testis.
- Secondary hydrocele.
- Lymphadenopathy (abdominal or cervical).
- Gynaecomastia.
- Symptoms due to metastases (e.g. backache).

**Investigations**

- Ultrasonography.
- Serum tumour markers ($\alpha$-fetoprotein, $\beta$-human chrionic gonadotrophin and lactate dehydrogenase).
- Orchidectomy (through inguinal approach) for histological examination.
- Staging investigations including CXR, CT (thorax and abdomen), lymphangiography, abdominal ultrasound and/or FNAC of extra-scrotal masses. The false negative rate for CT staging is 25%.

**Treatment and Prognosis**

- Stage I seminoma is treated by orchidectomy plus adjuvant chemo-therapy (1 or 2 courses of carboplatin) or radiotherapy. The disease free survival is 98–100%.
- Stage I non-seminoma is treated by orchidectomy plus nerve sparing retroperitoneal lymph node dissection (RPLND). Adjuvant chemo-therapy is given to patients with poor histological indicators (e.g. vascular invasion and anaplastic changes). The survival rate is 98% and relapse rate is 5%.
- Stage II seminoma is treated by radiotherapy or chemotherapy (carbo-plastin or etoposide/platinum).
- Stage II non-seminoma is treated by orchidectomy, RPLND and chemo-therapy (bleomycin/etoposide/platinum).
- Stage III/IV seminoma and non-seminoma are treated primarily with multiple courses of chemotherapy (bleomycin/etoposide/cisplatin). Surg-ical excision of metastases is performed in any patient with residual disease after tumour markers have been negative for more than 6 weeks. The primary cure rate is 85%.

# 45. Squamous Cell Carcinoma of the Penis

## Epidemiology

- It accounts for < 1% of all male cancers in the developed world.
- It is rare in males circumcised at birth or during childhood.

## Aetiology

- Circumcision prevents SCC of the penis.
- Premalignant lesions include Paget's disease, De Queryrat's erythro-plasia and Bowen's diseases of the glans penis.

## Pathology

- Stage I:   Tumour is confined to the glans or prepuce.
- Stage II:  Tumour involves penile shaft.
- Stage III: There is regional node involvement.
- Stage IV:  The nodes are fixed.

## Clinical Features

- An ulcer or reddened area on the glans.
- Purulent discharge.
- Inguinal lymphadenopathy.

## Investigations

- Surgical biopsy.
- FNAC of enlarged inguinal nodes.
- Pelvic CT for staging.

## Treatment

- Stage I is treated with radiotherapy (external beam or interstitial). If this fails, then partial penile amputation is performed.

- Stage II is treated with partial or total penile amputation. Perineal urethrostomy may be performed.
- Stage III is treated with radical phallectomy and regional lymphaden-opathy (one testis should be preserved).
- Stage IV may be palliated with toilet surgery.

## Prognosis

- The 5-year survival rate is 80% for well differentiated tumours and 20% for poorly differentiated ones.

# 46.  Primary Intracranial Tumours

## Epidemiology

- They occur in 4 per $10^5$ of the general population.
- The second commonest malignancy in children (after leukaemia).
- There are two peaks of incidence (1st decade and 5th/6th decades).

## Aetiology

- Genetic factors. CNS tumours are a major component of some inherited conditions such as tuberous sclerosis, neurofibromatosis and von-Hippel–Lindau syndrome.
- Radiation.
- Immunosuppression.

## Pathology

- According to cell origin, CNS tumours can be classified into glioma (the commonest type), medulloblastoma, neuroblastoma, meningioma, Schwannoma, neurofibroma and lymphoma.
- Gliomas include astrocytoma, oligodendroglioma, ependymoma and glioblastoma multiforme.

## Clinical Factors

- Symptoms and signs due to the local effects of the tumour on the surrounding structures which are destroyed and impaired due to infiltration, mechanical pressure and/or oedema.
- Symptoms and signs of raised intracranial pressure, e.g. headaches, vomiting and papilloedema.
- Shift of intracranial contents can cause compression of the brain stem and false localising signs.
- Seizures (complex, partial or simple).
- Progressive deterioration is the hallmark of clinical presentation.

**Investigations**

- MRI or CT scan.
- Skull X-rays are useful in pituitary and parasellar regions.
- Technetium brain scan may confirm the site of the lesion.
- Stereotactic or CT-guided biopsy.
- Other tests including an EEG, angiography and ventriculography.

**Treatment and Prognosis**

- Low-grade astrocytomas are treated by surgical excision followed by radiotherapy (external beam, interstitial or stereotactic) and chemotherapy (carmustine, lomustine, procarbine, cisplatin and vincristine).
- Ependymoma is treated with radiotherapy to the primary tumour site (50 Gy in 4–5 weeks). Craniospinal radiation is indicated for high-grade tumours. The overall 5-year survival rate is 40%.
- Oligodendroglioma is treated with surgical excision and post-operative radiotherapy. Chemotherapy is indicated for recurrent disease. The 10-year survival rate is 35%.
- Deep-seated gliomas are treated with radiotherapy (50 Gy in 4–5 weeks).
- Medulloblastoma is treated with surgical excision (if possible) and radiotherapy. The latter consists of brain irradiation down to the level of C2 (30 Gy in 3 weeks), a boosting dose to the posterior cranial fossa and mid-brain and spinal irradiation. Chemotherapy is indicated in young children and recurrent disease.
- Meningioma is treated with complete surgical excision. If this is not possible due to its location, then radiotherapy (55 Gy in 5–6 weeks) is used. This tumour is curable.
- Pituitary tumours are treated with trans-sphenoidal excision (if there is no supra-sellar extension) or excision through a craniotomy (if the tumour extends outside the pituitary fossa). Post-operative radiotherapy can be given. Prolactinomas may be treated with bromocriptine.
- Acoustic neuroma is treated by surgical excision.
- Seizures are treated with anticonvulsants, e.g. phenytoin.
- Cerebra oedema may be treated with corticosteroids (e.g. dexamethasone) and osmotic diuretic (e.g. mannitol or urea).
- Hydrocephalus can be treated with surgical decompression using ventriculo-peritoneal or ventriculo-atrial shunts.

# 47. Primary Spinal Cord Tumours

- Primary tumours of the spinal cord are uncommon.
- Ependymoma is the commonest tumour. Meningiomas and Scwannomas are relatively common whereas astrocytomas are rare.
- Treatment consists of high dose dexamethasone, surgical excision of the tumour (if possible) and post-operative radiotherapy. Spinal cord decompression should be performed (when indicated) even if the tumour is thought to be unresectable.

# 48. Cerebral Metastases

## Epidemiology

- 30% of patients with systemic cancer have cerebral metastases.
- The metastases are solitary in 50% and multiple in 50% of cases.

## Pathology

- The common primaries include breast, bronchus, melanoma, lymphoma and prostate.
- Spread is usually haematogenous.
- The metastasis is usually surrounded by cerebral oedema.
- Haemorrhage may occur within metastases, e.g. melanoma.

## Clinical Features

- Epilepsy, focal neurological deficit, raised intracranial pressure (ICP) and cerebellar symptoms and signs.

## Investigations

- MRI is the investigation of choice.
- Contrast-enhanced CT.
- Needle biopsy (under stereotactic guidance).
- Investigations of the primary lesion.

## Treatment

- Surgical excision is indicated for surgically accessible solitary metastases in the absence of apparent systemic disease in fit patients. Dexamethasone (4 mg qds for 2 days) and post-operative radiotherapy is given. The median survival rate is 2 years.
- Whole brain radiotherapy (35 Gy) and/or steroids for multiple metastases or surgically inaccessible lesions.

## Prognosis

- The overall median survival rate is 6 months.

# 49. Spinal Metastases

## Epidemiology

- Spinal metastases are found in 30% of patients dying of cancer.
- The thoracic spine is the commonest site.

## Pathology

- The common primaries include breast, bronchus, kidney, thyroid, prostate and haematological malignancies.
- Modes of spread include haematogenous (commonest), direct extension, perineural and lymphatic.
- Metastases may cause bony destruction, cord compression and deformity, spinal oedema, ischaemia and/or infarction.
- The metastases can be extradural (commonest), intradural/extramedullary or intradural/intramedullary.

## Clinical Features

- Pain (spinal or radicular).
- Urinary retention.
- Spastic paraplegia.
- Brown–Sequard's syndrome.
- Neurological symptoms and signs depending upon the degree of spinal involvement.

## Investigations

- FBC, erythrocyte sedimentation rate (ESR), LFTs, serum electrophoresis and serum biochemistry.
- CXR and plain radiographs of the spine.
- MRI is the investigation of choice.
- Myelography.
- CT (± myelography).
- CT-guided biopsy if the primary is unknown.
- Investigations for the primary lesion.

**Treatment**

- High-dose steroids to help with cord compression and oedema.
- Radiotherapy is effective in relieving cord compression and pain.
- Anterior spinal decompression or laminectomy is considered if there is neurological deterioration despite the radiotherapy and in relatively fit patients with a good prognosis; complete paraplegia lasting more than 24 hours is a contra-indication.
- The vertebral body can be reconstructed following anterior decompressing using methyl methacrylate and Steinmann's pins or iliac bone grafts.
- Posterior stabilisation of the spine may be performed following decompression.
- Anterior decompression can be performed through a thoracotomy, thoraco-abdominal retroperitoneal or transperitoneal approach, depending upon the site of compression.

# 50. Acute Leukaemia

## Epidemiology

- The incidence of acute myeloid leukaemia (AML) rises with age (15 per $10^5$ during the eighth decade).
- Acute lymphoblastic leukaemia (ALL) accounts for 80% of leukaemias during childhood (3 per $10^5$ during the first decade).
- AML accounts for 85% of leukaemias after the second decade.
- Male to female ratio is 3:2.

## Aetiology

- Ionising radiation.
- Benzene exposure.
- Cytotoxic chemotherapy.
- Occupational exposure, e.g. welding, DDT industries.
- Smoking increases the risk by 50%.
- Inherited syndromes, e.g. Down's syndrome, Bloom's syndrome, Fanconi's anaemia and ataxia telangiectasis.
- Specific chromosomal abnormalities, e.g. t(8;21) t(15;17) t(9;11) t(4;11), etc.
- Oncogene expression, e.g. C-fms in AML.
- Viruses.

## Pathology and Classification

*Morphological Classification of Acute Leukaemia*

- ALL:
    - $L_1$ Small monomorphic cells (scanty cytoplasm and fewer nucleoli).
    - $L_2$ Large heterogeneous cells (more common in adults).
    - $L_3$ Burkitt type.
- AML:
    - $M_1$ myeloblastic (no maturation).
    - $M_2$ myeloblastic (some maturation).
    - $M_3$ promyelocytic.
    - $M_4$ myelomonocytic.
    - $M_5$ monocytic.

- $M_6$ erythroleukaemia.
- $M_7$ megakaryoblastic.
- Cytochemical staining helps to determine the type of leukaemia in doubtful cases.
- Immunological classification of leukaemia helps in understanding the pathogenesis of the disease.

## Clinical Features

- ALL:
  - The symptoms include malaise, fever, bone pains, oral and pharyngeal ulceration and petechiae.
  - The signs include pallor, lymphadenopathy, hepatosplenomegaly, haemorrhages and bone tenderness. Mediastinal masses are more common in adults.
  - Symptoms and signs of malignant meningitis are occasionally present.
- AML:
  - The clinical features are similar to that of ALL.
  - Bone pain, lymphadenopathy and CNS involvement are less common than in ALL.
  - Gum hypertrophy is relatively common in $M_4$ and $M_5$.

## Investigations

- FBC may reveal anaemia, thrombocytopaenia and leukocytosis. Lymphoblasts or myeloblasts are usually present. The white blood cell (WBC) count may not be elevated.
- Bone marrow examination must show more than 30% of blast cells.
- Cytochemical staining and immunological typing is used when appropriate.
- Serum biochemistry.
- Clotting screen.
- CXR may show a mediastinal mass, especially in T-cell leukaemia, owing to thymic enlargement.
- Plain radiographs may show osteolytic lesions, demineralisation and/or radiolucent bands in the metaphysis.
- Lumbar puncture if indicated.

**Treatment**

- ALL:
  - Remission induction is achieved by vincristine, prednisolone and doxorubicin, followed by an intensive consolidation regimen consisting of doxorubicin, asparaginase, methotrexate and cytosine arabinoside.
  - CNS prophylaxis with cranial radiation (18 Gy in 10 fractions over 2 weeks) plus intrathecal methotrexate. CNS disease is treated by craniospinal radiation (24 Gy over 2 weeks).
  - Testicular disease is treated by radiation (24 Gy over 2 weeks).
  - Maintenance therapy for 2 years. Methotrexate, vincristine, prednisolone and mercaptopurine are used.
  - Relapse within the first year of treatment is an indication for bone marrow transplantation (BMT). Further intensive chemotherapy is indicated to reinduce remission in cases relapsing after 1 year of treatment.
  - BMT is also indicated in poor prognosis cases and in the second and third remission.
  - Allogenic BMT has a 5-year relapse-free survival rate of 65% in the second remission and a 3-year survival of 55% in the first remission.
  - Autologous BMT is also possible with less impressive results.
  - Treatment of adult ALL is similar to that of childhood ALL. However, the induction and maintenance treatments are more intense in view of the worse prognosis.
  - Supportive care includes blood and platelet transfusions, antimicrobials and allopurinol.
- AML:
  - Induction of remission with cytosine arabinoside, doxorubicin and 6-thioguanine. The mortality risk during induction is 10%.
  - Maintenance therapy includes cytosine arabinoside, cyclophosphamide, methotorexate, etoposide, 5-azacytidine and 6-mercaptopurine.
  - All-*trans*-retinoic acid (ATRA) is used in patients with $M_3$ to prevent DIC.
  - Supportive care includes blood and platelet transfusions, i.v. fluids, i.v. antimicrobials, haematopoietic growth factors, aseptic techniques in dealing with central venous catheters (e.g. Hickman line) and allopurinol.
  - Relapse is treated by reinduction chemotherapy or BMT.

**Prognosis**

- ALL:
  - The overall 5-year survival is 80% in girls and 50% in boys. The prognosis is worse in adults.

  AML:
  - The overall 10-year disease-free survival is 25%. Prognosis is worse in patients older than 30 years and with a high WBC.

# 51. Chronic Leukaemia

**Epidemiology**

- Chronic lymphocytic leukaemia (CLL) is a disease of the elderly.
- Chronic myelocytic leukaemia (CML) occurs in all age groups.

**Aetiology**

- See aetiology of acute leukaemia.
- Philadelphia chromosome (reciprocal translocation of part of the long arm of chromosome 22 to chromosome 9) occurs in most cases of CML.
- Trisomy of chromosome 12 and deletion 13q14 occur in CLL.

**Pathology**

- 95% of CLL cases are of the B-cell type. The T-cell type (5%) causes less immunoglobulin suppression and less lymphadenopathy. Auto-immune haemolytic anaemia occurs in 10% of CLL patients.
- Hypercellular bone marrow with lymphocytic or myeloid replacement.
- Infiltration of liver, spleen and lymph nodes.
- CLL can be staged into four stages depending upon the presence of anaemia, lymphadenopathy, splenomegaly and thrombocytopenia.

**Clinical Features**

- The patient may be asymptomatic.
- Symptoms include malaise, fatigue, weight loss, bruising and bleeding, abdominal discomfort, bone pains and fever.
- The signs include pallor, purpura, lymphadenopathy (especially in CLL), splenomegaly, hepatomegaly and signs of infection.

**Investigations**

- Blood count and film. In CLL lymphocyte count exceeds $10 \times 10^9$ litre$^{-1}$ (small well-differentiated lymphocytes). In CML there is leukocytosis with an increase in all granulocyte series, especially myelocytes.

Anaemia and thrombocytopenia are common.
* Bone marrow examination.
* Lymph node biopsy.
* Leukocyte alkaline phosphatase.


**Treatment**

* No treatment is indicated in asymptomatic patients. Blood counts are monitored regularly.
* Symptomatic patients with CLL are treated with chlorambucil (3 mg daily) until remission occurs. Relapse is treated with further chemotherapy. Other effective drugs include fludrabine and prednisolone. The latter is particularly useful in patients with bone marrow failure.
* Symptomatic patients with CML are treated with busulphan (70 mg/kg) until remission occurs (WBC $< 20 \times 10^9$/litre). Relapse is treated with further chemotherapy. Other effective drugs include hydroxyurea and $\alpha$-interferon.
* Blastic transformation of CML is treated appropriately as for AML and ALL.
* Allogenic BMT is considered during the first remission in patients with CML who are younger than 50 years and have a matched donor.
* Supportive care includes treatment of infections and transfusion of blood products (platelets and red blood cells).


**Prognosis**

* CLL:
    * The overall median survival is 5 years.
    * Poor prognostic indicators include lymphadenopathy, splenomegaly, anaemia and thrombocytopenia.
* CML:
    * The 5-year survival is less than 5%.
    * Allogenic BMT in suitable patients seems to cure 40% of patients, but long term results are awaited.
    * Philadelphia-negative type has a worse prognosis.


**Hairy Cell Leukaemia**

* This is regarded as a B-cell leukaemia.
* It is more common in males, especially during the 6th and 7th decades

of life.
- Anaemia, thrombocytopenia, neutropenia and splenomegaly are common features.
- Treatment modalities include α-interferon and 2-chlorodeoxyadenosine. The latter is becoming the drug of choice.

# 52. Hodgkin's Lymphoma

**Epidemiology**

- The incidence is approximately 1.8 per $10^5$ persons per year in Western countries. There is a geographical variation.
- The incidence gradually rises form the age of 10 years to reach a maximum at the age of 70 years. There is a fall during the 5th decade.
- The male to female ratio is 1.5:1.

**Aetiology**

- Familial tendency.
- The human leukocyte antigens (HLAs) HLA-A1 and HLA-A12 are both associated with the disease.
- Epstein–Barr virus genome can be detected in 40% of all cases.

**Pathology**

- Reed–Sternberg or mononuclear Hodgkin's cells are characteristic.
- Histological types:
  - Lymphocyte-depleted.
  - Lymphocyte-predominant.
  - Mixed cellularity.
  - Nodular sclerosis.
- The lymphocyte-predominant type has the best prognosis whereas the lymphocyte-depleted type carries a poor prognosis.

**Clinical Features**

- Lymphadenopathy. The neck is the most frequent site at presentation (70%) followed by axilla (20%) and groin (10%).
- Constitutional symptoms (fever, weight loss, pruritus and sweats) occur in 25% of patients. Alcohol-induced pain is reported in 3% of cases.
- Other features include autoimmune haemolytic anaemia, immune thrombocytopenia, erythema multiforme, erythroderma, lymphoderma, superior/inferior vena cava obstruction, obstructive jaundice, ureteric

obstruction and paraneoplastic syndromes.
- Hodgkin's disease may involve the spinal cord, lung, bone marrow, skin, gut, liver and/or spleen.

**Investigations**

- FBC, ESR and serum biochemistry.
- CXR (mediastinal and bronchopulmonary lymphadenopathy, thymus enlargement).
- Thoracic and abdominal CT.
- Biopsy (excisional or percutaneous).
- Other investigations include lymphangiography, bone marrow trephine and bone scan.
- Barium studies (if indicated).

**Ann Arbor Staging System**

- Stage I:   Involvement of a single node region or of a single extra lymphatic site or organ.
- Stage II:  Involvement of two or more node regions on the same side of the diaphragm.
            Involvement of a single extranodal site plus one (or more) node region on the same site of the diaphragm.
- Stage III: Involvement of lymph nodes on both sides of the diaphragm which may include the spleen or an extranodal site.
- Stage IV: Diffuse involvement of one or more extra lymphatic organs.
- A:        No constitutional symptoms.
- B:        Constitutional symptoms are present.

**Treatment**

- Stage IA and IIA: radiotherapy to the involved and adjacent lymph nodes (40 Gy in 20 fractions). Chemotherapy is reserved for relapse.
- Stage IIIA: combination chemotherapy, e.g. MOPP (mustine, oncovin, procarbazine and prednisolone), ABVD (adriamycin, bleomycin, vinblastine and decarbazine). Radiotherapy is used for residual and recurrent disease.
- Stage II B, III B and IV B: Combination chemotherapy.
- High-dose chemotherapy with stem cell support is indicated for extensive disease which fails to respond to standard chemotherapy regimens.

**Prognosis**

- The 10-year survival rates are:
    - 80% for stage IA.
    - 77% for stage IIA.
    - 72% for stage IIIA.
    - 65% for stage IIB.
    - 55% for stage IV.

# 53. Non-Hodgkin's Lymphoma (NHL)

## Epidemiology

- The incidence rises with age with a slight male predominance.
- There is a geographical variation in incidence and site. Burkitt's lymphoma (of the jaw) is common in Africa. Middle Eastern lymphoma usually effects the intestine.

## Aetiology

- Viruses: human T-cell leukaemia viruses HTLV1 and HTLV2, Epstein–Barr virus (EBV) and the herpes simplex virus HSV-6 have all been implicated.
- Immunosuppression, including congenital syndromes, and AIDS predispose to NHL.
- Coeliac disease predisposes to T-cell lymphoma of the intestine.
- Genetic factors – chromosomal translocation between chromosomes 8 and 14 and C-myc over-expression may contribute to aetiology.

## Pathology

- B-cell lymphoma (follicular, diffuse, Waldenström's, chronic lymphocytic leukaemia (CLL), Burkitt's lymphoma and heavy chain disease) accounts for 90% of cases.
- T-cell lymphoma (cutaneous thymic and peripheral cell lymphoma) accounts for 10% of cases.
- NHL can be classified in low grade, intermediate grade and high grade types.
- Immunological classification is helpful.

## Clinical Features

- Lymphadenopathy. The neck is the commonest site.
- Other clinical features include:
  - Hepatosplenomegaly.
  - Compression of structures, e.g. veins, ureters, hepatobiliary ducts, etc. and constitutional symptoms (fever, sweats and weight loss).

**Staging**

- This is the same as for Hodgkin's disease.
- Most patients have stage III or stage IV at presentation.

**Investigations**

- FBC and film, ESR, serum biochemistry.
- CXR. Thoracic and abdominal CT.
- Biopsy (excisional or percutaneous).
- Other investigations include; bone scan, lymphangiography and bone marrow trephine.
- Barium studies and IVU may be indicated.

**Treatment**

- Follicular lymphoma (40% of cases):
  - Stage I and II (small cell and mixed) disease is treated by radiotherapy to the involved and adjacent lymph nodes.
  - Stage I and II (large cell) disease is treated by radiotherapy and chemotherapy (CHOP regimen: cyclophosphamide, doxorubicin, vincristine and prednisolone).
  - Stage III and IV disease is treated with chemotherapy (low dose or high dose) and $\alpha$-interferon.
- Intermediate- and high-grade lymphoma (diffuse) is treated with combination chemotherapy (high dose).
- High-dose chemotherapy with peripheral stem cell support or autologous bone marrow transplantation for NHL unresponsive to standard regimens and for recurrent disease.
- Large-cell NHL in childhood is treated with an intensive induction course of chemotherapy followed by a consolidation phase and a maintenance course of alternating pairs of drugs.

**Prognosis**

- Follicular lymphoma. The 10-year survival is:
  - 78% for stage I.
  - 60% for stage II.
  - 52% for stage III.
  - 38% for stage IV.

- Diffuse intermediate and high-grade NHL. The 3-year disease free survival is 50%.
- Large NHL in childhood has a 5-year survival of 70% with modern management.
- Recurrent disease. The 3-year survival rate is 35% with high-dose chemotherapy.

# 54.  Multiple Myeloma

## Epidemiology

- The incidence is approximately 3 per $10^5$ persons per year. It rises with age.
- Males are more commonly affected.

## Pathology

- Infiltration of bone and bone marrow by malignant plasma cells causing osteoporosis, osteopenia, lytic lesions and pathological fractures.
- Paraproteinaemia (IgG, IgA, Bence–Jones, IgM and/or IgD) occurs in 99% of cases.
- Renal impairment (light chain deposition in the distal tabule, hyper-uricaemia, amyloidosis and hypercalcaemia).

## Clinical Features

- Diffuse bone pain is the commonest symptom (67%). Pathological fractures and cord compression may occur.
- Anaemia, recurrent infections, fatigue, nausea, and hypercalcaemia.
- Hyperviscosity syndrome.
- Hepatomegaly, splenomegaly and lymphadenopathy are uncommon.
- Other clinical features include: congestive cardiac failure and renal impairment.

## Investigations

- FBC, ESR, serum biochemistry and viscosity.
- Serum immunoglobulins and immunoelectrophoresis.
- $\beta_2$-microglobulin – plasma/urine.
- Bone marrow aspiration and trephine.
- 24 urinary light chains, proteins and calcium.
- Radiological skeletal survey.

## Treatment

- Serious complications, such as dehydration, hypercalcaemia and spinal cord compression, should be treated promptly with appropriate measures, e.g. fluid replacement, biphosphonates and radiotherapy to the spinal cord, etc.
- Combined melphalan–prednisolone oral therapy is the first line of treatment (6–9 courses). $H_2$ antagonists are usually added to therapy and α-interferon may be used as a maintenance therapy. The response rate is 60%. Some centres use more complex regimens of combination chemotherapy.
- Second-line chemotherapy includes agents such as doxorubicin, vincristine and nitrosoureas. Hemi-body irradiation is also effective as a second line therapy.
- Radiotherapy for painful bony deposits, spinal cord compressions and bones at risk of fracture.
- Internal fixation for pathological fractures and bones at risk.
- Supportive measures, e.g. blood transfusions and antibiotics.
- Monoclonal immunoglobulin levels can be used to monitor response to treatment.

## Prognosis

- Depends upon tumour mass:
  - The median survival is 5 years for low tumour mass, 2 years for intermediate tumour mass and 6 months for high tumour mass.

## Waldenström's Macroglobulinaemia

- There is production of monoclonal IgM and infiltration of bone marrow by lymphoid cells.
- The clinical features include hyperviscosity, weakness, haemolytic anaemia, purpura, bleeding disorders, hepatosplenomegaly and lymphadenopathy.
- The disease is slowly progressive and symptomatic cases require treatment in the form of oral chlorambucil or cyclophosphamide (small dose). Plasmapheresis is effective in reducing hyperviscosity.
- Multiple myeloma chemotherapy protocols can be used to treat aggressive disease.
- The median survival is 4 years.

# 55. Miscellaneous

### Carcinoma of the Maxillary Antrum

- It is usually diagnosed late after it has invaded surrounding structures.
- Unilateral nasal obstruction and blood-stained nasal discharge are early symptoms. The late clinical features include swelling of the cheek, swelling/ulceration of the palate or the bucco-alveolar sulcus, epiphora, proptosis, diplopia, pain and regional lymphadenopathy (submandibular and cervical).
- Systemic metastases are rare.
- The investigations include plain X-rays, CT and biopsy.
- The tumour is treated by a wide local excision (maxillectomy) combined with orbital exenteration if the orbit is involved, followed by radiotherapy.
- Unresectable tumours are treated by radiotherapy and chemotherapy.
- Management also includes reconstruction of surgical defects using temporalis muscle slings, skin grafts or composite bone flaps.
- The 5-year survival rate is 30%.

### Cancer of the Nasopharynx

- This type of cancer is relatively common in south China.
- Squamous cell carcinoma accounts for most cases. Lymphoma and adenoid cystic carcinoma are rare.
- The clinical features include nasal obstruction, blood-stained nasal discharge, cranial nerve palsies and cervical lymphadenopathy.
- Radiotherapy is the mainstay of treatment after three-dimensional radiation planning (up to 15 fields in a single patient). The neck is included in the radiation fields.
- Surgery is reserved for residual or recurrent disease.
- Chemotherapy is used for advanced disease in selected patients.
- The local control rate for T1 and T2 tumours is 90% compared with 45–75% for T3 and T4 tumours.

### Mesothelioma

- This is a malignant tumour of the pleura or pericardium.
- Pleural mesothelioma is strongly associated with blue (crocidolite) and

brown (amosite) asbestos. The latent interval between exposure and development of disease is approximately 30 years.
- The tumour tends to spread over the pleural surface encasing the lung and to invade the mediastinum, diaphragm and chest wall. A blood-stained pleural effusion is a common finding.
- Patients (aged 60 years) usually present with dyspnoea and chest pain.
- The investigations include CXR, CT, cytological analysis of pleural effusions, thoracoscopy and biopsy.
- Treatment is unsatisfactory. It includes surgical resection for localised lesions, radiotherapy and/or chemotherapy (systemic and/or intra-pleural). Cisplatin and α-interferon have a 20% response rate.
- Prognosis is poor with a median survival of 18 months from diagnosis.

## Chondrosarcoma

- This is the second commonest malignant tumour of bone. The pelvis is most commonly involved.
- The peak incidence occurs during 40–60 years of age.
- The disease may arise in benign enchondroma.
- Plain X-rays may show bone destruction and flecks of calcification. CT can demonstrate the extent of the lesion.
- Surgical excision of the lesion with endoprosthesis (if required) is the mainstay of management.
- Radiotherapy is used for palliation. Chemotherapy is occasionally used.

## Ewing's Sarcoma

- This is a malignant round cell tumour of bone with a peak incidence during the second decade of life.
- The pelvis and femur are most commonly affected.
- The clinical features include swelling, pain, fever, weight loss and dyspnoea due to pulmonary metastases.
- The investigations include plain X-rays, CT, MRI and biopsy.
- Treatment consists of radical radiotherapy combined with adjuvant chemotherapy (doxorubicin, cyclophosphamide, vincristine, actinomycin D and ifosfamide).
- The 5-year survival for patients with localised disease is 55%.

## Cutaneous T-Cell Lymphoma ('Mycosis Fungoides')

- The peak incidence occurs during the fifth and sixth decades of life. The sex distribution is equal.
- The disease has four stages:
  - Stage I:    Plaque or eczematous skin lesions.
  - Stage II:   Plaque with enlarged lymph nodes which are pathologically negative.
  - Stage III:  Erythroderma.
  - Stage IV:   Visceral enlargement of pathologically positive nodes.
- Sézary syndrome is a form of disseminated disease.
- Treatment modalities include PUVA, wide field radiation, whole body electron therapy and/or chemotherapy (alkylating agents and interferon).

## Merkel Cell Tumour

- This is a rare primary cutaneous neuroendocrine tumour.
- It usually presents as a discrete nodular mass.
- The tumour is primarily treated by radiotherapy (90% response rate) or surgery with a 72% survival at 2 years.

## Uveal Melanoma

- The incidence is 6 per $10^6$ per year. It is the commonest intraocular malignancy in adults.
- 85% of lesions arise in the choroidal part, the remainder (13%) arise in the ciliary body and iris.
- The clinical features include a visual field defect, pain, secondary glaucoma and retinal detachment. Systemic metastases are common.
- Treatment modalities include photocoagulation, cryotherapy, radiotherapy and/or surgery.
- The indications for enucleation include pain, secondary glaucoma, invasion of surrounding structures and macular/optic nerve involvement.

## Squamous Cell Carcinoma of the Bladder

- Accounts for 3% of all bladder cancers.
- Risk factors include:
  - Chronic infection, e.g. schistoma haematobium cystitis.
  - Stones.

- Long-term catheterisation and neuropathic bladders.
- The disease is usually advanced at presentation.
- The tumour is treated by radical cystectomy.
- The tumour is not radiosensitive.

### Neuroblastoma

- Arises from adrenal or neural crest tissue.
- Occurs in 1 of every 10 000 live births.
- The clinical features include abdominal mass, neurological signs and symptoms, Horner's syndrome and distant metastases (liver, skin and bone).
- The investigations include bone marrow aspiration, urinary, VMA, CXR, FBC, serum biochemistry, bone scan, USS, CT and/or MRI.
- Treatment consists of surgical debulking and adjuvant radiotherapy. Other treatment modalities include chemotherapy and autologous bone marrow transplantation.
- Prognosis depends on stage, age, location, site of metastases, presentation and the presence of the N-myc oncogene.
- The overall survival rate varies between 10% and 90% depending on the stage of the disease.

# 56.  Long-term Venous Access

## Indications

- Administration of cytotoxic drugs.
- Total parental nutrition (TPN).
- Transfusion of blood products.
- Administration of antimicrobials.
- Bone marrow or peripheral stem cell infusion.

## Catheters

- These are usually made of silicone (low thrombogenicity and flexibility) or polyurethane.
- They can be single, double or triple lumen. The last-mentioned is associated with a higher incidence of sepsis.
- Hickman lines are wide-bore silicone catheters which were described in 1979. Groshing lines are similar to Hickman lines but have self-sealing valves to prevent reflux of blood into the line.

## Insertion Techniques

- Catheters can be inserted using a surgical cut-down technique or a percutaneous (Seldinger) introducer kit.
- The procedure can be performed under general or local anaesthesia.
- The internal jugular, subclavian, external jugular and cephalic veins are usually selected for cannulation. The inferior vena cava is occasionally selected, e.g. superior vena cava (SVC) obstruction.
- The operating table is tilted head down to allow distension of veins and prevent air embolism.
- The catheter tip should lie at the right atrium/SVC junction or in the SVC. X-ray control is used to confirm the catheter position.
- The catheter should be tunnelled subcutaneously so that the exit point is approximately 15 cm down the chest wall. Tunnelling helps line stabilisation and reduces the infection risk.
- A Dacron cuff is positioned near the skin exit site and the induced fibrosis helps stabilisation of the line.
- Totally implantable devices have parts or reservoirs with a self-sealing silicone septum, e.g. Port-Cath.
- Totally implantable pumps are also available.

**Complications**

- Sepsis:
  - Skin exit site infection requires dressing and antimicrobials, e.g. vancomycin.
  - Tunnel infection requires catheter removal.
  - Catheter/tip infection responds to vancomycin if due to *S. epidermidis* – removal is frequently required.
- Pneumothorax incidence should be < 3%.
- Air embolism.
- Injury of neighbouring structures during catheter insertion.
- Catheter fracture.
- Catheter occlusion can be treated with heparin or streptokinase (250 000 units).
- Vein thrombosis.
- Extravasation of drugs can occur with totally implantable devices.


**Principles of Catheter Care**

- Aseptic technique.
- Flushing with heparin/saline once weekly if the catheter is not in regular use. Totally implantable devices may be flushed once monthly.
- Nurse's training.
- Patient's education.

# 57. Pain Control in Advanced Cancer

- Pain is a complex symptom with sensory and emotional components. Its severity should be decided by the patient and not the carer.
- Empathy, good communication skills and regular assessment are essential to pain management.
- The cause of pain should be accurately diagnosed and removed if possible.
- The analgesic is chosen in a stepped approach (the analgesic ladder) which consists of:
  - Step 1 Non-opioids, e.g. paracetamol 1 g 6-hourly, Ibuprofen 200–600 mg 8-hourly, diclofenac 50 mg 8-hourly, Entonox, nefeopam, etc.
  - Step 2 Weak opioids, e.g. codeine and dihydrocodeine.
  - Step 3 Strong opioids, e.g. morphine, diamorphine (for subcutaneous route) and Fentanyl (for transdermal administration).
- The starting dose of strong opioids depends upon the previous analgesic needs and on renal function. Hepatic dysfunction has a limited clinical impact on opiate metabolism.
- Secondary analgesia relieves pain through an indirect mechanism. They include antidepressants (e.g. amitriptyline, lofepramine), corticosteroids, antispasmodics (e.g. hyoscine butylbromide), carbamazepine, sodium valproate and membrane stabilising drugs.
- Spinal analgesia via an intrathecal catheter (strong opioid/bupivacaine mixture) has a role in patients unable to tolerate the adverse effects of systemic opioids.
- Peripheral nerve blocks may be also used in pain control.
- The management of bone metastases also includes radiotherapy, orthopaedic fixation of pathological fractures, biphosphonates (e.g. clodronate), nerve block and hormonal manipulation where appropriate.
- Neurosurgical procedures for pain control, e.g. cordotomy for unilateral pain are occasionally required and liaison with neurosurgical colleagues is needed.

# 58. Symptom Control in Advanced Cancer

- Pain is a complex symptom with sensory and emotional components. Its severity should be decided by the patient and not the carer (see Section 57).
- Nausea and vomiting:
  - The choice of an antiemetic depends upon the cause. A single antiemetic is sufficient in most cases.
  - The cause, e.g. hypercalcaemia, should be specifically treated if appropriate.
  - Antihistamines such as cyclizine and hyoscine hydrobromide are effective in the treatment of vomiting due to stimulation of vomiting centres.
  - Potent dopamine antagonists such as haloperidol are effective in the treatment of vomiting due to stimulation of chemoreceptor trigger zone.
  - Peripheral dopamine antagonists such as metoclopramide and domperidone are effective against vomiting due to gastric stasis.
  - Other antiemetics used include ondansetron (serotonin antagonists) and cisapride (gastrointestinal stimulant).
  - Associated management of nausea and vomiting include dexamethasone and nasogastric drainage and percutaneous gastrostomy.
- Dysphagia:
  - Malignant dysphagia can be relieved by oesophageal intubation, radiotherapy, laser or dexamethasone.
  - Viral infections and candidiasis causing dysphagia should be appropriately treated, e.g. fluconazole, Zovirax, etc.
  - Hydration and feeding can be achieved via gastrostomy.
  - The swallowing therapist may play an important role.
- Bowel obstruction:
  - The causes include recurrent abdominal tumour, metastatic obstruction, a primary tumour, constipation, benign adhesions and ileus.
  - Surgery should be considered in fit patients with obstruction suspected to be due to a single site obstruction or benign adhesions provided the patient is willing to undergo surgery.
  - Hyoscine is used to relieve colics.
  - Most patients will absorb sufficient fluid from their upper GI tract to prevent symptomatic dehydration. Parenteral nutrition is only indicated in the pre-operative preparation for surgery.
- Diarrhoea:

- Causes such as constipation, infection, partial bowel obstruction, carcinoid syndrome and postgastrectomy syndrome should be considered.
- The management includes rehydration and loperamide.
- The management of steatorrhoea includes loperamide, ranitidine, pancreatin supplement and/or biliary drainage (bypass surgery or endoscopic stenting).
- Blind-loop syndrome can be treated with antibiotics, e.g. tetracycline, metronidazole.
- Radiotherapy – induced diarrhoea responds to NSAIDs.
- Octreotide is used for severe refractory diarrhoea.
- Constipation:
  - It should be prevented in high risk patients by regular use of co-danthrusate 2 capsules at night. The laxative dose is titrated according to the opiate dose in order to maintain comfortable stools.
  - If the rectum is full, constipation is treated with glycerine suppositories and phosphate enemas. If unsuccessful, manual evacuation under sedation should be considered.
  - Other drugs used in the treatment of constipation include bisacodyl (10–20 mg po or pr) and docusate (100–300 mg tds).
- Oral problems:
  - Oral hygiene is essential.
  - Aphthous ulceration is treated with tetracycline.
  - Suspension and topical corticosteroids.
  - Fungal infections are treated with fluconazole (a single dose) and nystatin suspension.
  - Benzydamine hydrochloride (Difflam) mouthwash provides effective oral analgesia.
- Anorexia:
  - Can be helped with corticosteroids (e.g. dexamethasone 4 mg daily) or megestrol (160 mg daily).
- Ascites:
  - The commonest causes of malignant ascites are carcinomas of the bronchus, breast, stomach, pancreas, colon and ovary.
  - Paracentesis offers immediate relief and can be achieved using a peritoneal dialysis catheter inserted through the left iliac fossa or the mid line suprapubically under local anaesthesia. The ascites is drained to dryness over 6 hours and a colostomy bag is placed over the puncture site.
  - Spironolactone combined with frusemide helps long-term control.
  - Peritoneo-venous shunt (Le-Veen shunt) can be inserted under a general anaesthetic in suitable patients.
- Pleural effusions:

- Pleural effusions are worth draining if symptomatic (1.5 litres at a time). If the effusion recurs, the pleurodesis with 1 g of tetracycline is indicated after drainage to dryness through an intercostal drain. Talc powder achieves a 100% control rate but causes a vigorous reaction.
- Pleuroperitoneal shunt is a recognised treatment modality in selected patients.
- Anxiety and depression:
  - Anxiety is relieved by empathy, explanation, counselling and relaxation.
  - Depression (early morning wakening, self-blame, worthlessness and loss of interest) can be effectively treated with antidepressants, e.g. amitriptyline (75–150 mg daily) and lofepramine (140–210 mg daily).